I0757380

Menopause

Hot Flashes & Cool Wisdom

A Survival Guide with Practical Tips, Humor, and Self-Care for Thriving Through Menopause.

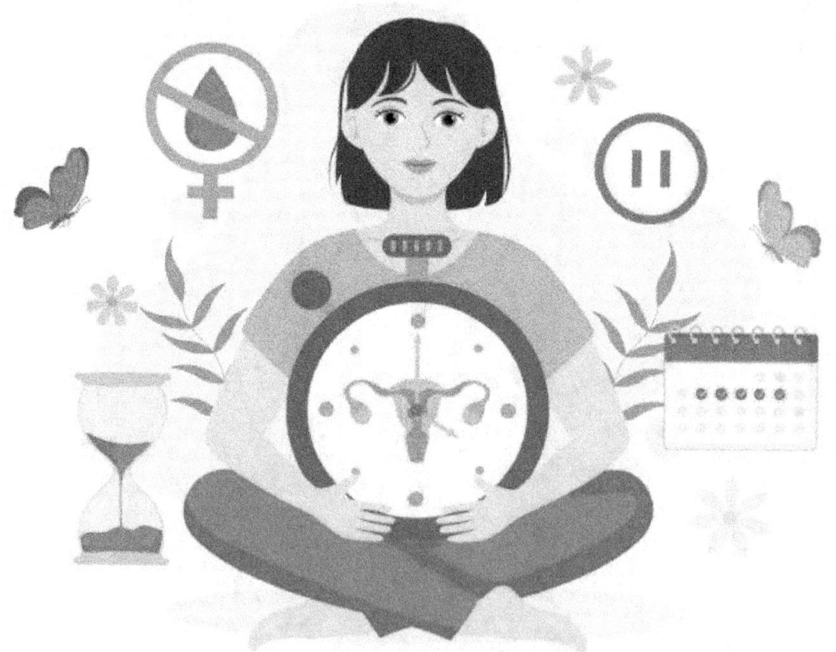

Menopause: Hot Flashes & Cool Wisdom

A Survival Guide with Practical Tips, Humor, and Self-Care for Thriving Through Menopause.

Written by Sophie Lynn

Contents

Introduction

Welcome to the New Chapter of Life

Menopause is a transformative stage in every woman's life, marking the end of menstruation and the beginning of a new chapter. While this transition can come with a variety of physical and emotional changes, it is also a time for renewal and empowerment. In this introduction, we'll explore the basics of what's happening in your body, how to embrace the changes with humor and grace, and why the "survival guide" approach—packed with practical tips, humor, and self-care—is key to thriving during menopause.

Understanding Menopause: What's Happening to My Body?

Menopause is a natural biological process that occurs when a woman's ovaries produce less estrogen and progesterone, leading to the end of menstruation. While this process is a normal part of aging, the symptoms and experiences vary greatly among women, both in intensity and duration.

The Stages of Menopause

- **Perimenopause**: This is the transition phase leading up to menopause, usually starting in a woman's 40s but sometimes earlier. During this time, hormone levels fluctuate, causing irregular periods, mood swings, and symptoms such as hot flashes.

- **Menopause**: Officially marked when a woman has not had a menstrual period for 12 consecutive months, typically occurring between the ages of 45 and 55. The ovaries significantly decrease hormone production during this stage.

- **Postmenopause**: This follows menopause and lasts for the rest of a woman's life. While some symptoms of menopause may subside, the lower hormone levels can increase risks for certain health conditions, such as osteoporosis and heart disease.

Common Symptoms of Menopause

- **Hot Flashes and Night Sweats**: Sudden warmth in the upper body, often accompanied by redness and sweating, are common during menopause. Night sweats are the nighttime version, often leading to sleep disturbances.

- **Mood Swings and Irritability**: Fluctuations in hormone levels can lead to emotional ups and downs, making you feel fine one moment and anxious or irritable the next.

- **Weight Gain and Slower Metabolism**: The hormonal changes can cause shifts in body fat distribution and a slower metabolism, making it harder to maintain or lose weight.

- **Vaginal Dryness**: As estrogen levels drop, vaginal tissues can become drier and less elastic, leading to discomfort during intercourse.

- **Sleep Problems**: Insomnia, waking up frequently, or having trouble falling asleep are common issues during menopause.

While these symptoms can seem daunting, understanding them is the first step in managing them. Menopause is a significant change, but it doesn't mean you have to suffer through it.

Embracing the Change with Humor and Grace

Many women dread menopause because it represents the end of youth and fertility, but this mindset doesn't have to define your experience. Menopause is just another phase of life—one that can be met with humor, grace, and even optimism.

Finding the Humor in Menopause

Menopause can be funny! Yes, hot flashes in the middle of a business meeting or waking up drenched in sweat aren't ideal, but laughing at these moments can make them less stressful. Here are some ways to embrace the humor:

- **Hot Flash Funnies**: Treat hot flashes like impromptu workouts. "Hey, who needs a sauna when your body's got its own heating system?" Recognize that others may find your sudden fan-flapping and open-window requests amusing—and laughter can defuse tension.

- **Mood Swings**: The unpredictability of emotions during menopause is real, but instead of getting frustrated, find the humor in being able to cry over commercials one moment and laugh at them the next. Remind yourself (and others) that it's just hormones.

- **Forgetfulness**: "Menopause brain" can lead to moments where you forget why you walked into a room or what you were about to say. Instead of getting embarrassed, laugh it off—everyone has these moments eventually, and menopause just speeds up the timeline.

Grace in Acceptance

Menopause can sometimes feel like a loss, especially when it comes to the end of fertility, but it can also be a time of growth, self-reflection, and empowerment. Rather than fighting the changes, embrace them as part of the natural aging process:

- **Redefine Beauty**: Society often equates youth with beauty, but this is a perfect time to challenge those standards. Midlife can be the most confident, radiant period of your life—when you are more comfortable in your skin and wiser from life's experiences.

- **Acceptance of the New Normal**: Gracefully accepting that your body is going through changes can reduce the stress of trying to control things outside your power. Recognize that menopause is a normal part of life, not a deficiency or problem to be fixed.

- **Celebrating a New Phase**: Many women feel liberated after menopause because they no longer have to deal with monthly periods, PMS, or the possibility of pregnancy. There's a newfound freedom in knowing you've reached a significant milestone.

The Survival Guide Approach: Practical Tips, Humor, and Self-Care

The "Hot Flashes & Cool Wisdom" survival guide approach combines practical strategies, humor, and self-care to help you not only survive but thrive through menopause.

Practical Tips

- **Managing Hot Flashes**: Wear light, breathable fabrics, and dress in layers so you can remove them when a hot flash strikes. Keep a small fan or cooling spray handy for emergencies. Avoid hot beverages, spicy foods, and alcohol, which can trigger hot flashes.

- **Sleep Solutions**: Create a calming bedtime routine to combat sleep disturbances. Lower the temperature in your bedroom, invest in moisture-wicking sheets, and try relaxation techniques like deep breathing or meditation before bed.

- **Dealing with Mood Swings**: Regular exercise, a balanced diet, and mindfulness can help stabilize mood swings. Engage in activities that bring you joy and relaxation, whether it's yoga, painting, or spending time with friends.

Humor as a Coping Tool

- **Create a Menopause Playlist**: Fill it with funny and empowering songs to lighten your mood. Songs like "Hot Stuff" by Donna Summer or "I'm Still Standing" by Elton John can bring a smile to your face when you need it most.

- **Join a Community**: Surround yourself with women going through similar experiences. Sharing funny stories and anecdotes with others who "get it" can help lighten the emotional load.

Self-Care Strategies

- **Nurturing Yourself**: Now is the time to focus on self-care. Whether it's taking long baths, scheduling regular massages, or indulging in hobbies you love, nurturing your mental and physical well-being should be a priority.

- **Healthy Lifestyle Choices**: Menopause is a good time to reassess your diet and exercise habits. Focus on nutrient-dense foods, especially those rich in calcium and vitamin D, to support bone health. Incorporate strength training to counteract muscle loss and stay active.

- **Mindfulness and Meditation**: Practicing mindfulness or meditation can help reduce stress and improve your emotional well-being. A few minutes of mindful breathing each day can have a significant impact on managing menopause symptoms.

Why This Book? The Power of Information, Support, and Laughter

This book isn't just a medical manual—it's a guide to living well through menopause. By arming yourself with information, embracing humor, and creating a strong support system, you can manage menopause with grace and positivity. Here's why this book will be your companion on the journey:

- **Information is Power**: The more you know about what's happening to your body, the better equipped you'll be to manage symptoms and make informed health decisions.

- **Laughter is Healing**: Humor helps lighten the burden of menopause. It allows you to step back, laugh at the absurdity of it all, and not take the challenges so seriously.

- **Support is Key**: You don't have to go through menopause alone. This book encourages you to seek out support—whether from loved ones, health professionals, or communities of women who understand what you're going through.

Part I: The Basics of Menopause

Chapter 1

What Exactly is Menopause?

Menopause is a natural part of aging, but its onset, symptoms, and duration can vary significantly from one woman to another. In this chapter, we'll explore the different phases of menopause, the hormonal changes driving it, common myths, and the various timelines and factors that influence when it starts. Understanding these foundational concepts is key to navigating this life stage with confidence and clarity.

Menopause

Menopause is officially defined as the point in time when a woman has not had a menstrual period for 12 consecutive months. It marks the end of her reproductive years. On average, menopause occurs between the ages of 45 and 55, though it can happen earlier or later depending on genetic, lifestyle, and health factors.

Perimenopause

Perimenopause refers to the transitional period leading up to menopause, during which a woman's body begins to produce less estrogen and progesterone. This stage can last anywhere from a few months to several years and is typically characterized by irregular periods, hormonal fluctuations, and the onset of menopausal symptoms such as hot flashes, mood swings, and sleep disturbances.

- **Key Symptoms of Perimenopause:**
    - Irregular periods (may be heavier, lighter, or more spaced out)
    - Hot flashes and night sweats
    - Mood swings, irritability, or anxiety
    - Changes in libido

    o   Vaginal dryness or discomfort during intercourse

Postmenopause

Postmenopause begins after a woman has gone 12 months without a menstrual period. During this phase, many symptoms of menopause may continue but often decrease in intensity over time. However, the long-term effects of reduced estrogen levels—such as increased risks for osteoporosis, heart disease, and urinary issues—become more prominent. This stage lasts for the rest of a woman's life, and maintaining overall health through diet, exercise, and regular medical check-ups is crucial.

The Hormonal Roller Coaster: Estrogen, Progesterone, and Beyond

The hallmark of menopause is the fluctuation and eventual decline of key hormones, particularly **estrogen** and **progesterone**. These hormones play critical roles in regulating the menstrual cycle, mood, and bodily functions, so their reduction leads to many of the symptoms associated with menopause.

Estrogen

Estrogen is one of the main female sex hormones and is responsible for regulating the menstrual cycle, supporting bone density, maintaining vaginal and skin health, and contributing to the functioning of the cardiovascular system. As estrogen levels decline during menopause, women often experience:

- Hot flashes

- Night sweats

- Vaginal dryness

- Reduced bone density, increasing the risk of osteoporosis

- Increased risk of heart disease

Progesterone

Progesterone works alongside estrogen to regulate the menstrual cycle and support pregnancy. During perimenopause, progesterone production decreases, leading to irregular periods and changes in bleeding patterns. Low progesterone can also contribute to sleep issues and mood swings.

Other Hormones

- **Testosterone**: Though typically considered a male hormone, women also produce testosterone, which helps regulate libido and energy levels. Testosterone production decreases during menopause, contributing to lower sex drive and reduced energy.

- **Follicle-Stimulating Hormone (FSH)**: As estrogen production falls, the body compensates by producing more FSH, which stimulates the ovaries. Rising FSH levels are often used as an indicator of approaching menopause.

The dramatic shifts in these hormones can make menopause feel like an emotional and physical roller coaster. However, understanding these changes can help you manage the transition more effectively.

Menopause Myths: Debunking Common Misconceptions

There are many misconceptions about menopause, some of which can cause unnecessary anxiety or confusion. Let's clear up a few of the most common myths.

Myth 1: Menopause Happens Overnight

While the official definition of menopause refers to a single point in time—the 12-month mark after your last period—the transition into menopause, known as **perimenopause**, can last several years. During this time, your hormones fluctuate, and you may experience various symptoms. Menopause is a gradual process, not an immediate event.

Myth 2: Menopause Only Affects Older Women

While menopause typically occurs between ages 45 and 55, some women experience early menopause (before age 40), known as **premature menopause**. This can be due to genetics, autoimmune diseases, or medical treatments like chemotherapy. Additionally, women who have had a hysterectomy or oophorectomy (removal of ovaries) may experience **surgical menopause** earlier than the typical age range.

Myth 3: Menopause is the End of Your Sex Life

While menopause can cause vaginal dryness and reduced libido due to hormonal changes, it doesn't mean the end of a fulfilling sex life. Many women find that with the right treatments (e.g., lubricants, vaginal moisturizers, hormone therapy), they can maintain or even improve their sexual health during and after menopause. Open communication with a partner and healthcare provider can also help address these concerns.

Myth 4: Hormone Therapy is Dangerous for Everyone

Hormone Replacement Therapy (HRT) is often misunderstood. While there are risks associated with HRT, especially for women with certain medical conditions, it can be highly effective for many women in managing menopausal symptoms. Advances in HRT options mean treatments can be customized to your specific health needs, so it's important to consult with your healthcare provider about your options.

Myth 5: All Women Experience the Same Symptoms

Menopause affects each woman differently. Some women have few symptoms, while others may experience more severe physical and emotional changes. Genetics, lifestyle, and health history all play a role in determining how a woman experiences menopause. There is no "one-size-fits-all" experience.

When Does It Start? Timelines and Variability

The timing of menopause is influenced by several factors, including genetics, health, and lifestyle choices. While there is no exact formula for determining when you'll experience menopause, understanding the variability can help set realistic expectations.

The Average Age of Menopause

Most women reach menopause between the ages of **45 and 55**, with the average age being around 51. However, factors like family history, smoking, and medical conditions can influence the timing.

- **Genetics**: If your mother or sisters experienced menopause at a particular age, you might too. Genetics play a significant role in determining the timing of menopause.

- **Smoking**: Women who smoke tend to experience menopause 1-2 years earlier than non-smokers, as smoking can accelerate the depletion of eggs in the ovaries.

- **Health Conditions**: Autoimmune diseases, thyroid disorders, or certain medical treatments (e.g., chemotherapy) can lead to earlier menopause.

Perimenopause: The Early Warning Signs

Perimenopause often starts in a woman's **40s** but can begin as early as the mid-30s for some women. This phase lasts for an average of 4 to 8 years, during which hormone levels fluctuate and menopausal symptoms start to appear. During perimenopause, periods may become irregular, heavier, or lighter, and women may begin to experience hot flashes, night sweats, and mood swings.

Early or Premature Menopause

For some women, menopause begins earlier than expected, either due to medical conditions or surgical procedures.

- **Premature Menopause** occurs before the age of 40 and can be caused by genetics, autoimmune diseases, or certain medical treatments like chemotherapy.

- **Surgical Menopause** happens when a woman has both ovaries removed (oophorectomy), often due to conditions like endometriosis or ovarian cancer.

Postmenopause: Life After Menopause

Postmenopause refers to the years after menopause, and while some symptoms like hot flashes may diminish, others—like increased risk for osteoporosis and heart disease—become more significant. Maintaining a healthy lifestyle during this phase is crucial for long-term well-being.

Understanding menopause means knowing that it's not just a single event but a series of stages involving complex hormonal changes. From perimenopause through postmenopause, each woman's experience is unique. By learning the facts, debunking myths, and recognizing the variability of menopause timelines, you can approach this new chapter with confidence and preparedness. In the upcoming chapters, we'll dive deeper into managing the symptoms, maintaining your health, and embracing the opportunities this phase of life offers.

Chapter 2

Menopause 101: Understanding the Symptoms

Menopause brings with it a host of physical and emotional changes, many of which can be frustrating and confusing. In this chapter, we'll explore the most common symptoms of menopause, why they occur, and practical strategies for managing them. From hot flashes to weight gain, understanding what's happening in your body will help you navigate this transition with more control and confidence.

Hot Flashes: Why They Happen and How to Cool Down

Hot flashes are one of the most well-known and disruptive symptoms of menopause. These sudden, intense feelings of heat often start in the chest and face, then spread throughout the body. They can last anywhere from 30 seconds to several minutes and are sometimes followed by chills as your body tries to regulate temperature.

Why Do Hot Flashes Happen?

Hot flashes are caused by the fluctuating and decreasing levels of **estrogen** during menopause. The hypothalamus, which controls body temperature, becomes more sensitive to slight changes. When estrogen levels drop, the hypothalamus can falsely detect that your body is too hot, triggering a hot flash. This leads to the widening of blood vessels near the skin (causing flushing), sweating, and an increased heart rate.

- **Triggers for Hot Flashes**:

    o Spicy foods

    o Caffeine

    o Alcohol

    o Stress

    o Warm environments (e.g., hot rooms, direct sunlight)

How to Cool Down

While hot flashes can't always be prevented, there are several ways to reduce their frequency and intensity:

- **Dress in Layers**: Wear lightweight, breathable clothing and layer so that you can remove clothing as you feel a hot flash coming on.

- **Stay Cool**: Use fans or cooling sprays to quickly lower your body temperature. Keep ice water nearby, and avoid hot drinks.

- **Watch Your Diet**: Avoid common hot flash triggers like caffeine, alcohol, and spicy foods. Instead, focus on a diet rich in plant-based estrogens (phytoestrogens) such as soy, flaxseed, and tofu.

- **Try Relaxation Techniques**: Stress can exacerbate hot flashes, so practice deep breathing, meditation, or yoga to help calm your nervous system.

- **Hormone Therapy (HRT)**: For women experiencing severe hot flashes, hormone replacement therapy may be recommended by a healthcare provider. HRT can help regulate estrogen levels, reducing the frequency and severity of hot flashes.

Symptoms of Menopause: A Comprehensive Guide

Menopause is a natural biological process marking the end of a woman's reproductive years. It is characterized by the cessation of menstrual periods and is often accompanied by a variety of physical and emotional symptoms due to hormonal fluctuations, primarily the decline of estrogen and progesterone. This guide explores the common symptoms of menopause, their impact on daily life, and practical solutions to manage them.

Common Symptoms of Menopause

1. Hot Flashes

Overview:

- Hot flashes are sudden feelings of warmth that can spread throughout the body, often accompanied by sweating and sometimes chills.

- They can occur at any time of the day or night and can last from a few seconds to several minutes.

Solutions:

- **Lifestyle Changes:**

    - **Dress in Layers:** Wearing layers can help you adjust your body temperature more easily.

    - **Avoid Triggers:** Identify and avoid triggers such as spicy foods, alcohol, caffeine, and stress.

- **Cooling Techniques:**

    - **Use Fans or Air Conditioning:** Keep your environment cool.

    - **Cool Showers:** Taking cool showers can help lower your body temperature during an episode.

- **Mind-Body Techniques:**

    o **Deep Breathing Exercises:** Practice deep breathing to help calm your body and mind when a hot flash strikes.

2. Night Sweats

Overview:

- Night sweats are episodes of excessive sweating that occur during sleep, often leading to disrupted sleep and discomfort.

Solutions:

- **Sleep Environment:**

    o **Choose Breathable Fabrics:** Use moisture-wicking sheets and pajamas to help regulate temperature during the night.

- **Hydration:**

    o **Stay Hydrated:** Drink plenty of water throughout the day, especially before bed, to maintain hydration levels.

- **Medication:**

    o **Discuss with Your Doctor:** If night sweats severely disrupt sleep, consult a healthcare provider about possible treatments, including hormone therapy or non-hormonal medications.

3. Vaginal Dryness

Overview:

- Vaginal dryness occurs due to decreased estrogen levels, leading to thinning and drying of the vaginal tissues, which can cause discomfort during intercourse.

Solutions:

- **Lubricants and Moisturizers:**

    o **Water-Based Lubricants:** Use during intercourse to reduce friction.

- o **Vaginal Moisturizers:** Apply regular vaginal moisturizers to alleviate dryness.

- **Hormonal Treatments:**

    - o **Local Estrogen Therapy:** Consult a healthcare provider about vaginal estrogen creams, tablets, or rings that can help restore moisture in the vaginal area.

4. Mood Swings

Overview:

- Hormonal changes during menopause can lead to mood swings, irritability, and heightened emotions, which may mimic premenstrual syndrome (PMS).

Solutions:

- **Mindfulness and Stress Management:**

    - o **Meditation and Yoga:** Incorporate mindfulness practices to help manage stress and improve emotional regulation.

- **Physical Activity:**

    - o **Regular Exercise:** Engage in regular physical activity to boost endorphins and improve mood.

- **Cognitive Behavioral Therapy (CBT):**

    - o **Therapeutic Support:** Consider therapy to develop coping strategies for managing mood swings.

5. Weight Gain

Overview:

- Many women experience weight gain during menopause, often due to metabolic changes, hormonal fluctuations, and lifestyle factors.

Solutions:

- **Healthy Eating:**

  - **Balanced Diet:** Focus on whole foods, including fruits, vegetables, whole grains, lean proteins, and healthy fats to support metabolism.

- **Regular Exercise:**

  - **Strength Training:** Incorporate strength training into your routine to build muscle mass and boost metabolism.

  - **Cardiovascular Activity:** Aim for at least 150 minutes of moderate aerobic activity weekly to help manage weight.

6. Fatigue

Overview:

- Fatigue is a common complaint during menopause, which can result from sleep disturbances, hormonal changes, and emotional stress.

Solutions:

- **Prioritize Sleep:**

  - **Sleep Hygiene:** Establish a relaxing bedtime routine and maintain a consistent sleep schedule.

- **Balanced Lifestyle:**

  - **Nutrition and Hydration:** Ensure a balanced diet and adequate hydration to support energy levels.

- **Limit Caffeine and Alcohol:**

  - **Avoid Stimulants:** Reduce intake of caffeine and alcohol, especially in the evening, to improve sleep quality.

Emotional and Psychological Effects

The hormonal changes during menopause can significantly impact mental health, leading to increased risks of anxiety and depression. Here's how:

1. Hormonal Impact on Mental Health

- **Estrogen and Mood Regulation:** Estrogen plays a role in the production of serotonin and other neurotransmitters that regulate mood. Lower levels can contribute to feelings of sadness or anxiety.

- **Stress and Life Changes:** The transition into menopause often coincides with other life changes, such as aging parents, empty nesting, or career shifts, which can exacerbate emotional challenges.

2. Strategies for Emotional Well-Being

- **Professional Support:**

    - **Therapy:** Consider seeking help from a mental health professional to address anxiety, depression, or mood swings. Cognitive-behavioral therapy (CBT) can be particularly effective.

- **Support Groups:**

    - **Peer Support:** Join a menopause support group to connect with others experiencing similar challenges, providing an opportunity to share experiences and coping strategies.

- **Mindfulness and Relaxation Techniques:**

    - **Meditation and Breathing Exercises:** Incorporate mindfulness techniques into your daily routine to reduce stress and promote emotional balance.

- **Physical Activity:**

    - **Regular Exercise:** Engage in regular physical activity to boost mood and combat fatigue.

Menopause is a natural transition that comes with various physical and emotional symptoms. Understanding these symptoms and their implications can empower women to seek effective management strategies. By adopting a holistic approach that includes lifestyle changes, medical options, and emotional support, women can navigate this transition with resilience and grace. Remember, you are not alone in this journey, and seeking support from healthcare providers, friends, and family can make a significant difference in your experience of menopause.

Mood Swings and Emotional Changes: It's Not Just in Your Head

The emotional roller coaster that comes with menopause can be just as challenging as the physical symptoms. Many women experience mood swings, irritability, anxiety, and even depression during this transition. These emotional changes are linked to hormonal fluctuations, particularly with estrogen and progesterone, which also affect brain chemistry.

Why Mood Swings Happen

Estrogen has a significant impact on the production of **serotonin**, a neurotransmitter that helps regulate mood. As estrogen levels decline, serotonin production can drop, leading to feelings of irritability or sadness. Additionally, the stress of coping with physical symptoms, such as hot flashes and sleep disturbances, can take a toll on emotional well-being.

- **Common Emotional Symptoms:**
    - Irritability
    - Anxiety or nervousness
    - Sadness or depression
    - Difficulty concentrating (sometimes referred to as "menopause brain")
    - Feeling overwhelmed or stressed by minor issues.

How to Manage Emotional Changes

- **Stay Active**: Exercise is one of the most effective ways to boost your mood. Physical activity increases the production of endorphins, which help improve your emotional state. Even a 30-minute walk can make a big difference.

- **Mindfulness and Meditation**: Practicing mindfulness or meditation can help you manage stress and reduce anxiety. Breathing exercises can calm the mind and help you regain emotional balance.

- **Talk It Out**: Don't hesitate to share your feelings with trusted friends, family, or a therapist. Sometimes just acknowledging what you're going through can lift a significant emotional burden.

- **Consider Supplements**: Some women find relief from mood swings with supplements like **St. John's Wort, black cohosh**, or **evening primrose oil**. However, it's important to discuss these options with a healthcare provider to ensure they're safe for you.

- **Hormone Therapy**: As with hot flashes, HRT can help stabilize hormone levels and alleviate mood swings for some women.

Sleep Disruptions: Battling Insomnia and Night Sweats

Many women going through menopause experience **insomnia, night sweats**, or general sleep disturbances. Whether you have trouble falling asleep, staying asleep, or are awakened by sudden sweating episodes, these disruptions can make menopause feel even more overwhelming.

Why Sleep Problems Happen

- **Night Sweats**: Like daytime hot flashes, night sweats occur when estrogen fluctuations affect your body's ability to regulate temperature, often causing you to wake up drenched in sweat.

- **Insomnia**: Hormonal changes can interfere with sleep cycles. The drop in estrogen affects the production of **melatonin**, the hormone responsible for regulating sleep. Additionally, stress and anxiety associated with menopause can lead to difficulty relaxing and falling asleep.

- **Frequent Urination**: Menopause can also lead to changes in the bladder, resulting in more frequent trips to the bathroom at night, further disrupting sleep.

How to Improve Sleep

- **Create a Cool Sleep Environment**: Keep your bedroom cool and comfortable. Use a fan or air conditioning, and consider moisture-wicking sheets or pajamas to help absorb sweat.

- **Establish a Sleep Routine**: Going to bed and waking up at the same time every day can help regulate your sleep cycle. Avoid using screens (phones, tablets) before bed, as the blue light can interfere with melatonin production.

- **Cut Back on Stimulants**: Reduce caffeine, especially in the afternoon and evening, and limit alcohol, as both can worsen sleep disruptions.

- **Relaxation Techniques**: Try deep breathing, meditation, or progressive muscle relaxation before bed. These techniques can help calm your mind and prepare your body for sleep.

- **Hormone Therapy**: If night sweats or insomnia are severely affecting your quality of life, talk to your healthcare provider about whether HRT or other medications might help.

Weight Gain and Metabolism Shifts: Why Does My Body Feel Different?

Weight gain during menopause is a common concern for many women. The combination of a slower metabolism, changes in fat distribution, and hormonal shifts can lead to extra pounds—particularly around the abdomen.

Why Weight Gain Happens

During menopause, the body's metabolism slows down due to hormonal changes, specifically the reduction in estrogen. Estrogen helps regulate body fat distribution, and as levels drop, many women notice fat accumulating around the midsection. Additionally, the loss of muscle mass that often accompanies aging can make it harder to burn calories, contributing to weight gain.

- **Changes in Fat Distribution**: Menopausal women often experience a shift in where their body stores fat. Whereas pre-menopause fat may have been distributed more evenly, post-menopause fat tends to accumulate around the abdomen, increasing the risk of metabolic issues such as heart disease and type 2 diabetes.

How to Manage Weight Gain

- **Strength Training**: Incorporating weight-bearing exercises or resistance training can help you maintain muscle mass and boost metabolism. Building muscle increases the number of calories your body burns at rest.

- **Prioritize Protein**: A diet rich in lean protein can support muscle maintenance and help control hunger. Include foods like eggs, chicken, fish, legumes, and nuts in your meals.

- **Watch Portion Sizes**: With a slower metabolism, you may need fewer calories than before. Be mindful of portion sizes, and focus on whole, nutrient-dense foods like vegetables, fruits, whole grains, and lean proteins.

- **Stay Active**: Incorporating physical activity, even in small ways like walking or taking the stairs, can help you manage weight and improve your overall health.

- **Mindful Eating**: Pay attention to hunger cues and avoid emotional eating, which can become more common as mood swings and stress take hold. Techniques like mindful eating can help you stay in tune with your body's needs.

- **Hydration**: Drink plenty of water throughout the day. Staying hydrated helps manage hunger and can prevent overeating.

Menopause can introduce a range of challenging symptoms, from hot flashes and mood swings to weight gain and sleep disruptions. However, by understanding what's happening in your body and adopting practical strategies, you can manage these changes and maintain a sense of control. In the next chapters, we'll explore more self-care strategies, lifestyle changes, and humor-filled ways to embrace this new phase of life with resilience and grace.

Chapter 3

Navigating the Doctor's Office

Managing menopause often involves regular visits to your healthcare provider, where you'll discuss symptoms, treatment options, and overall health. This chapter will guide you on what to expect at your doctor's visit, the role of Hormone Replacement Therapy (HRT), important lab tests, and key questions to ask to ensure you're making informed decisions about your health.

What to Expect at Your Doctor's Visit

When you visit your healthcare provider to discuss menopause, it can be helpful to know what to expect so that you can make the most of your appointment. Whether you're experiencing perimenopause, menopause, or postmenopause, your doctor will focus on your symptoms, medical history, and long-term health.

Discussing Your Symptoms

Your doctor will ask about the frequency, intensity, and duration of your symptoms. Be prepared to discuss:

- **Hot flashes and night sweats**

- **Mood changes** (such as irritability or anxiety)

- **Sleep disruptions** and any issues with insomnia

- **Changes in your menstrual cycle** (if still in perimenopause)

- **Vaginal dryness** or discomfort during intercourse

- **Weight changes** or other body changes

- **Sexual health** and libido changes Tracking these symptoms in a journal before your visit can be helpful to provide an accurate overview.

Medical History and Family History

Your healthcare provider will review your medical history, including any chronic conditions, surgeries, or medications you're taking. They'll also ask about your family history, particularly regarding menopause, osteoporosis, heart disease, and cancers like breast and ovarian cancer. These factors will help determine the best approach to managing your menopause symptoms and overall health.

Physical Exams

Depending on your symptoms and health status, your doctor may perform several physical exams, including:

- **Pelvic exam** to check the health of your reproductive organs.

- **Breast exam** to screen for abnormalities or signs of breast cancer.

- **Bone density test** (especially if you're at risk for osteoporosis).

- **Blood pressure check** and other cardiovascular screenings.

Understanding what to expect can reduce anxiety and ensure you make the most of your visit by discussing any concerns.

Hormone Replacement Therapy (HRT): Pros, Cons, and Alternatives

Hormone Replacement Therapy (HRT) is one of the most commonly discussed treatments for managing menopause symptoms, particularly hot flashes, night sweats, and vaginal dryness. However, it's essential to weigh the pros and cons and explore alternatives before deciding if it's right for you.

What is HRT?

HRT involves supplementing your body with estrogen (and sometimes progesterone) to compensate for the natural decline of these hormones during menopause. It can be taken in various forms, including pills, patches, gels, or vaginal creams.

Types of HRT

- **Estrogen-only HRT**: Prescribed for women who have had a hysterectomy (removal of the uterus).

- **Combination HRT**: Includes both estrogen and progesterone, often prescribed for women who still have their uterus to reduce the risk of endometrial cancer.

The Pros of HRT

- **Relief from Hot Flashes and Night Sweats**: HRT is highly effective in reducing the frequency and intensity of hot flashes and night sweats.

- **Improved Vaginal Health**: It can alleviate vaginal dryness, itching, and discomfort during intercourse by restoring moisture and elasticity to vaginal tissues.

- **Prevention of Osteoporosis**: HRT helps maintain bone density, reducing the risk of fractures and osteoporosis.

- **Mood Stability**: Some women find that HRT improves mood swings and helps with sleep by stabilizing hormone levels.

The Cons of HRT

- **Increased Risk of Certain Cancers**: Long-term HRT, especially combination HRT, has been associated with an increased risk of breast cancer and endometrial cancer. The risks depend on the length of time HRT is used and individual factors.

- **Cardiovascular Risks**: HRT can increase the risk of blood clots, strokes, and heart disease, particularly in older women or those with pre-existing conditions.

- **Other Side Effects**: Some women may experience side effects such as bloating, breast tenderness, or headaches while on HRT.

Alternatives to HRT

If HRT isn't suitable for you or you prefer not to take it, there are several non-hormonal options available:

- **Lifestyle Changes**: Regular exercise, a balanced diet, and stress reduction techniques like yoga and meditation can help alleviate symptoms.

- **Medications**: Certain antidepressants (SSRIs) have been shown to reduce hot flashes and mood swings. Other medications, like gabapentin, may help with night sweats.

- **Vaginal Moisturizers and Lubricants**: Over-the-counter products can address vaginal dryness without the need for hormone therapy.

- **Herbal Supplements**: Some women find relief with supplements such as **black cohosh**, **soy isoflavones**, or **red clover**, though scientific evidence on their effectiveness is mixed. Always consult your doctor before trying supplements.

Lab Tests and What They Tell You About Your Health

Certain lab tests can provide important insights into your hormonal levels, bone health, and cardiovascular risks as you transition through menopause. These tests can guide treatment decisions and help monitor your overall health.

Hormone Levels

Your doctor may order tests to check your levels of:

- **Follicle-Stimulating Hormone (FSH)**: Elevated FSH levels are a common indicator that you're approaching menopause, as your ovaries stop responding to FSH.

- **Estrogen**: As estrogen declines during menopause, measuring your levels can help determine if HRT or other treatments may be beneficial.

- **Thyroid Function**: Thyroid issues can mimic menopause symptoms, so checking your thyroid hormones can rule out conditions like hypothyroidism.

Bone Density Test (DEXA Scan)

A **bone density test** measures the strength of your bones and is particularly important for postmenopausal women, who are at increased risk for osteoporosis due to declining estrogen levels. This test helps assess your fracture risk and whether you may need medications or lifestyle changes to protect your bone health.

Cholesterol and Blood Sugar

Menopause increases the risk of cardiovascular disease due to changes in fat distribution and metabolic health. Your doctor may order:

- **Lipid Panel**: To check your cholesterol levels. High LDL (bad cholesterol) and low HDL (good cholesterol) levels increase the risk of heart disease.

- **Blood Glucose Levels**: To monitor for diabetes or prediabetes, which can become more common during and after menopause.

Other Lab Tests

Depending on your symptoms and health history, your doctor may recommend additional tests, such as **liver function tests** (especially if you're considering HRT) or **iron levels** if you've been experiencing fatigue or anemia.

Questions to Ask Your Healthcare Provider

Your doctor's visit is an opportunity to get clear on your health and treatment options. Here are key questions to ask during your visit:

About Symptoms and Menopause Stages:

1. How do I know if I'm in perimenopause, menopause, or postmenopause?

2. Are my symptoms typical for menopause, or could they indicate another health issue?

3. What lifestyle changes can help reduce my symptoms?

About Treatment Options:

1. What are the risks and benefits of HRT for someone with my medical history?

2. Are there non-hormonal treatments that can help manage my hot flashes, mood swings, or other symptoms?

3. How long would I need to be on HRT, and when should I consider stopping it?

About Lab Tests:

1. Which tests will you order, and what information will they give us about my health?

2. Do I need a bone density test or other screening tests at this stage of menopause?

About Long-Term Health:

1. How does menopause affect my risk for osteoporosis, heart disease, and other conditions?

2. What can I do now to protect my bone and cardiovascular health as I age?

Navigating the doctor's office during menopause doesn't have to be daunting. By understanding the purpose of your visit, the pros and cons of treatments like HRT, and the importance of lab tests, you can take an active role in managing your health. Don't hesitate to ask questions and explore options with your healthcare provider to find the best path for you. In the next chapters, we'll delve deeper into self-care strategies and how to handle menopause with humor, grace, and resilience.

Part II: Thriving Through the Transition

Chapter 4

Mastering Hot Flashes with Cool Strategies

Hot flashes are one of the most common and challenging symptoms of menopause. They can come on suddenly, disrupting your day or night with a rush of heat, sweat, and discomfort. While you can't eliminate hot flashes entirely, you can manage them effectively with a combination of short-term cooling techniques and long-term lifestyle adjustments. In this chapter, we'll explore practical strategies to keep you cool, comfortable, and in control.

Quick Cool-Down Techniques: Breathing, Water, and Ice Packs

When a hot flash strikes, it's important to have immediate tools at hand to cool down quickly. These strategies offer fast relief and can help you regain your composure, whether you're at work, home, or out in public.

1. Deep Breathing

Focused, deep breathing can calm your body's response during a hot flash by reducing stress and helping to regulate body temperature.

- **How It Works**: Slow, deep breaths signal to your nervous system to relax, which can reduce the intensity of a hot flash.

- **Technique**: Inhale slowly for a count of four, hold for four, then exhale for a count of four. Repeat this cycle until the hot flash subsides.

2. Water

Drinking cool water or splashing your face with water can quickly lower your body temperature.

- **Tip**: Keep a bottle of cold water with you at all times. Drinking small sips throughout the day can also prevent dehydration, which can worsen hot flashes.

3. Ice Packs and Cooling Towels

For immediate relief, use cold compresses or cooling towels to lower your body temperature.

- **Tip**: Store small ice packs or cooling towels in your freezer. If you're on the go, use a portable fan or cooling wristbands to help dissipate heat.

Long-Term Solutions: Diet, Exercise, and Supplements

While quick fixes are essential for in-the-moment relief, adopting long-term lifestyle changes can help reduce the frequency and severity of hot flashes over time.

1. Diet and Hydration

The foods and drinks you consume play a significant role in how your body handles temperature regulation. Some foods can trigger hot flashes, while others can help keep you cool.

- **Avoid Triggers**: Common hot flash triggers include spicy foods, alcohol, caffeine, and high-sugar foods. Reducing or eliminating these from your diet may help reduce hot flashes.

- **Eat Cooling Foods**: Incorporate more fresh fruits, vegetables, and whole grains into your diet. Foods rich in phytoestrogens, such as soy, flaxseeds, and tofu, may help balance hormone levels.

- **Stay Hydrated**: Drink plenty of water throughout the day to stay cool and hydrated. Aim for at least eight glasses a day, more if you're active or live in a warm climate.

2. Exercise and Physical Activity

Regular exercise can help regulate your body's temperature, reduce stress, and improve your overall well-being.

- **Focus on Aerobic Exercise**: Activities like walking, swimming, or cycling help improve circulation, which can prevent your body from overheating.

- **Strength Training**: Building muscle mass helps boost metabolism and maintain a healthy weight, both of which can reduce the frequency of hot flashes.

- **Relaxation Exercises**: Mind-body practices like yoga and tai chi can help reduce stress and lower the intensity of hot flashes through breathing and mindfulness techniques.

3. Supplements

Some natural supplements may help balance hormones or reduce the severity of hot flashes.

- **Black Cohosh**: A popular herbal remedy for hot flashes, though its effectiveness can vary from person to person.

- **Soy Isoflavones**: Soy-based supplements can mimic the effects of estrogen, potentially reducing hot flashes in some women.

- **Evening Primrose Oil**: This supplement is sometimes used to alleviate hot flashes, though results can be mixed. Always consult your healthcare provider before starting any supplement regimen to ensure it's safe for you.

Dressing for Success: Fabrics and Clothing Choices to Beat the Heat

The clothes you wear can make a significant difference in how your body handles temperature changes during a hot flash. Smart wardrobe choices can help you stay cool and comfortable throughout the day.

1. Opt for Breathable Fabrics

Lightweight, natural fabrics like cotton, linen, and bamboo are breathable and allow your skin to cool down faster than synthetic fabrics like polyester.

- **Cotton and Linen**: These fabrics are breathable and wick away moisture, making them ideal for managing sweat during hot flashes.

- **Moisture-Wicking Fabrics**: If you're active or tend to sweat a lot, opt for moisture-wicking workout clothes designed to keep you cool during physical activities.

2. Layering

Dressing in layers allows you to easily adjust your clothing as your body temperature changes throughout the day.

- **Strategy**: Wear a lightweight tank top or t-shirt under a cardigan or jacket. You can remove layers as needed when a hot flash starts, and then add them back on once it passes.

3. Choose Comfortable, Loose-Fitting Clothes

Tight clothing can trap heat and make a hot flash feel more intense. Opt for loose-fitting garments that allow air to circulate.

- **Tip**: Flowing dresses, wide-leg pants, and loose-fitting tops are great options for staying cool while still looking stylish.

4. Nightwear and Bedding

Hot flashes can disrupt your sleep, especially if you're not wearing the right nightwear or using heavy bedding.

- **Lightweight Pajamas**: Choose moisture-wicking or lightweight cotton pajamas that won't trap heat.

- **Cooling Bedding**: Use cotton or bamboo sheets, and consider a cooling pillow or mattress topper to help regulate your temperature at night.

Creating a Hot-Flash Emergency Kit

Having a hot-flash emergency kit on hand can provide peace of mind and quick relief when you're out and about. This kit is easy to assemble and can fit in your purse, car, or desk drawer.

What to Include in Your Kit

1. **Cooling Towel**: A compact, portable cooling towel that activates with water can provide immediate relief.

2. **Portable Fan**: A small, battery-operated fan can help you cool down quickly in any situation.

3. **Water Bottle**: A refillable water bottle is essential for staying hydrated throughout the day.

4. **Face Mist or Cooling Spray**: A cooling spray or facial mist can instantly refresh your skin and lower your body temperature.

5. **Extra Layers**: A lightweight cardigan or wrap you can take off during a hot flash.

6. **Ice Pack or Cooling Wristbands**: Small, portable gel packs or wristbands designed to lower your body's core temperature.

How to Use Your Kit

- **At Work**: Keep your kit in your desk drawer for easy access during meetings or work tasks.

- **In Public**: If you feel a hot flash coming on, use the cooling spray, fan, or ice pack to cool down quickly and discreetly.

- **At Night**: Keep a smaller version of your kit by your bedside for easy access to water, a fan, or a cooling towel to help you get back to sleep faster after a night sweat.

Mastering hot flashes involves a combination of quick cooling techniques, long-term lifestyle adjustments, and being prepared for unexpected moments. By incorporating these strategies into your daily routine, you'll feel more in control and less overwhelmed by hot flashes. In the next chapter, we'll explore how to manage mood swings and emotional changes with resilience and self-compassion, helping you stay balanced throughout menopause.

Chapter 5

Finding Humor in the Heat: Laughing Through Menopause

Menopause can be a challenging time, filled with unexpected symptoms and emotional ups and downs. However, finding humor in these experiences can be a powerful tool for coping and thriving during this transition. In this chapter, we'll explore how embracing the lighter side of menopause can help you navigate the journey with a smile, share real-life stories from women who've been there, and delve into the science behind how laughter positively impacts your health.

Funny Moments: Finding the Lighter Side of Menopause

Embracing humor during menopause doesn't mean ignoring the challenges; rather, it's about acknowledging them and choosing to see the amusing aspects. Laughing at the absurdities can lighten your mood, reduce stress, and even bring you closer to others who share similar experiences.

1. The Surprise Sauna Experience

Imagine standing in the frozen food aisle at the grocery store when, suddenly, you feel like you're in a sauna. You're fanning yourself with a box of waffles while fellow shoppers look on in confusion. Instead of feeling embarrassed, picture yourself saying, "Well, who needs a tropical vacation when you have menopause?"

Tip: Keep a hand-held fan or a folding paper fan in your purse. Not only is it practical, but it can also be a conversation starter, allowing you to share a laugh with others.

2. The Case of the Disappearing Glasses

Have you ever searched high and low for your reading glasses, only to realize they're perched atop your head? Menopause can bring about moments of forgetfulness, often referred to humorously as "menopause brain."

Funny Anecdote: One woman recounted how she once tore apart her entire house looking for her car keys, only to find them in the refrigerator next to the milk. Instead of frustration, she chuckled and said, "At least my keys were staying cool!"

3. Mood Swings and Family Antics

Mood swings can be unpredictable, but sometimes they lead to hilariously over-the-top reactions that, in hindsight, are more amusing than upsetting.

Example: After bursting into tears because her favorite TV show was a rerun, a woman laughed with her family about how "even the television is experiencing mood swings!"

4. Fashion Faux Pas Turned Fun

Waking up drenched from night sweats might lead you to wear mismatched socks or your shirt inside out. Rather than feeling self-conscious, own it with humor.

Suggestion: When someone points out the mishap, you might say, "I'm just starting a new fashion trend—didn't you get the memo?"

5. The Unpredictable Thermostat

Your internal thermostat might be on the fritz, but that can lead to some amusing situations. If you're bundled up in a sweater one minute and fanning yourself the next, use it as an opportunity for a light-hearted joke.

Quip: "Welcome to the menopausal weather channel: today's forecast is hot with a chance of cold flashes!"

Hormonal Hijinks: Real-Life Stories from Women in the Trenches

Hearing from other women who've navigated menopause can be both comforting and entertaining. Their stories remind us that we're not alone and that there's plenty to laugh about along the way.

1. The Board Meeting Blush

Story: Linda, a 52-year-old executive, was in the middle of a critical board meeting when a hot flash hit. Feeling the heat rising, she decided to address it head-on: "Ladies and gentlemen, if you notice me turning red, it's not from the numbers on page five—it's just my personal summer kicking in!" The room erupted in laughter, easing the tension and making the meeting more enjoyable.

Lesson: Embracing and acknowledging what's happening can diffuse awkwardness and create a shared moment of levity.

2. The Case of the Phantom Menopause Symptoms

Story: Maria kept experiencing strange symptoms—tingling in her fingers, sudden bouts of laughter, and an uncontrollable urge to dance when she heard music. Worried, she visited her doctor, who assured her that these were just her body's unique responses to hormonal changes. Relieved, Maria embraced these quirks, jokingly referring to herself as "Menopause's Got Talent."

Lesson: Accepting and finding joy in your body's changes can transform worry into amusement.

3. The Great Grocery Store Escape

Story: During a particularly intense mood swing, Sophie felt overwhelmed in the grocery store and abandoned her cart in the aisle. Later, she laughed with friends, saying, "Some people do a mic drop; I do a cart drop!"

Lesson: Sharing these stories with friends can turn a frustrating experience into a humorous anecdote.

4. The Night Sweat Chronicles

Story: Carol woke up one night feeling like she had swum across the Atlantic. Instead of getting upset, she changed into her husband's oversized t-shirt and announced, "I've decided to take up midnight swimming—no pool required!"

Lesson: A playful attitude can make inconvenient symptoms more bearable.

5. The Memory Lane Mishap

Story: After forgetting her best friend's birthday, Janet felt terrible but decided to make light of it. She sent a belated birthday card that read, "I'm not late; I'm just on menopause time!"

Lesson: Using humor to address forgetfulness can ease any embarrassment and keep relationships strong.

The Power of Humor: How Laughter Can Help You Cope

Humor is more than just entertainment; it's a valuable coping mechanism that offers physical and emotional benefits, especially during menopause.

1. Physical Benefits of Laughter

- **Stress Reduction:** Laughter decreases stress hormones like cortisol and adrenaline, helping to relax your body.

- **Immune System Boost:** It increases the production of antibodies and activates immune cells, improving your resistance to illness.

- **Pain Relief:** Laughter triggers the release of endorphins, the body's natural painkillers.

Example: Joining a laughter yoga class combines the benefits of physical exercise with the healing power of laughter, enhancing your overall well-being.

2. Emotional and Mental Health Advantages

- **Mood Enhancement:** Laughing elevates your mood, making it easier to cope with anxiety or irritability.

- **Social Connection:** Sharing laughs with others strengthens relationships and reduces feelings of isolation.

- **Perspective Shift:** Humor allows you to see situations from a different angle, reducing the intensity of negative emotions.

Tip: Watch comedies, read humorous books, or follow funny social media accounts to incorporate more laughter into your daily routine.

3. Strategies to Cultivate Humor

- **Keep a Humor Journal:** Write down funny incidents or thoughts. Revisiting these entries can lift your spirits during challenging times.

- **Surround Yourself with Lighthearted People:** Spend time with friends or family members who make you laugh.

- **Don't Take Yourself Too Seriously:** Give yourself permission to be silly or playful. Embrace the imperfect moments—they often make the best stories.

Exercise: Try standing in front of the mirror and making funny faces or reciting tongue twisters. It might feel ridiculous, but that's the point!

4. Laughter as a Stress Management Tool

- **Laughter Meditation:** Start with a gentle smile and allow it to grow into a hearty laugh. Even forced laughter can lead to genuine amusement.

- **Humorous Affirmations:** Create positive, funny affirmations like, "I'm not losing my memory; I'm making room for more important things!"

Case Study: A study published in the *Journal of Women's Health* found that women who incorporated daily laughter reported a significant reduction in menopausal symptoms compared to those who didn't.

5. Incorporating Humor into Daily Life

- **Decorate with Whimsy:** Place humorous quotes or cartoons around your home or workspace.

- **Share the Laughter:** Send funny memes or jokes to friends experiencing menopause. It builds camaraderie and mutual support.

- **Attend Comedy Events:** Go to stand-up shows or improv nights. Being in an environment focused on laughter can be invigorating.

Finding humor during menopause isn't about minimizing the challenges; it's about empowering yourself to handle them with resilience and joy. Laughter offers a respite from discomfort, strengthens connections with others, and enhances your physical and emotional health. By embracing the funny moments, sharing stories, and actively seeking out humor, you transform menopause from a period of struggle into an opportunity for growth and happiness.

Remember, every hot flash, mood swing, or forgetful moment carries the potential for a good laugh. So, the next time you find yourself in an awkward or frustrating menopausal moment, ask yourself, "How can I find the humor in this?" You might be surprised at how a little laughter can make the heat a bit more bearable.

Action Steps:

1. **Start a Humor Collection:** Gather jokes, stories, or quotes that make you laugh, and refer to them when you need a mood boost.

2. **Connect with Others:** Join a support group or online community where women share humorous menopause experiences.

3. **Practice Laughter Daily:** Set aside time each day to engage in activities that make you laugh, whether it's watching a funny video or chatting with a friend.

4. **Share Your Stories:** Don't hesitate to share your own menopausal mishaps with others—they might just brighten someone else's day.

By infusing your menopause journey with humor, you not only cope better with the changes but also enrich your life and the lives of those around you. So go ahead—laugh through menopause and embrace the power of humor to heal and uplift.

Chapter 6

Mind Over Menopause: Emotional Well-Being and Mental Health

As menopause brings significant changes to your body, it also affects your emotional and mental well-being. Hormonal fluctuations can lead to mood swings, anxiety, irritability, and even depression. But menopause is not just about managing symptoms—it's also an opportunity for personal growth and emotional clarity. This chapter will explore practical strategies for maintaining emotional balance, incorporating self-care routines, and embracing menopause as a time of renewal and reinvention.

Dealing with Mood Swings: Practical Tips for Emotional Balance

Mood swings during menopause are often triggered by hormonal changes, particularly the fluctuating levels of estrogen and progesterone. These can cause feelings of irritability, sadness, or anxiety seemingly out of nowhere. While these emotional highs and lows can feel overwhelming, there are ways to manage them effectively and regain your sense of balance.

1. Recognize the Triggers

Understanding what might be triggering your mood swings is the first step in managing them. Hormonal shifts are the root cause, but other factors—like stress, lack of sleep, or certain foods—can exacerbate these fluctuations.

- **Track Your Moods:** Keeping a mood journal can help you identify patterns. Note the days you feel especially irritable or emotional and try to connect them to specific events, foods, or lifestyle choices.

- **Common Triggers:** Caffeine, alcohol, processed foods, and lack of sleep are often culprits in worsening mood swings. Pay attention to your diet and sleep schedule to help manage your emotions.

2. Practice Emotional Awareness

When you feel a mood swing coming on, pause and acknowledge what you're feeling without judgment. Recognizing your emotions gives you the opportunity to respond to them in a healthy way, rather than letting them control you.

- **Breathe Through It:** Take a few deep breaths to calm your mind and body. Try the 4-7-8 breathing technique: inhale for 4 seconds, hold for 7, and exhale for 8.

- **Name Your Emotions:** By identifying and labeling your emotions (e.g., "I feel frustrated" or "I'm overwhelmed"), you can better understand what's driving them and respond more calmly.

3. Communicate Your Feelings

If mood swings are affecting your relationships, it's important to communicate openly with loved ones about what you're going through.

- **Be Honest:** Let your partner, family, or friends know that mood swings are a normal part of menopause, and sometimes you may need space or understanding.

- **Ask for Support:** Don't hesitate to ask for help or a listening ear when you're feeling emotionally overwhelmed. Talking through your feelings can reduce the intensity of mood swings.

4. Physical Activity as an Emotional Outlet

Exercise is a powerful tool for stabilizing emotions and releasing tension.

- **Aerobic Exercise:** Activities like walking, running, or swimming help release endorphins, the body's natural mood lifters, reducing feelings of anxiety and depression.

- **Yoga or Tai Chi:** These mind-body practices combine movement with breathing techniques, promoting relaxation and emotional balance.

Self-Care Routines for Mental Clarity

Menopause can sometimes bring about "brain fog," where you might feel forgetful, unfocused, or mentally sluggish. Creating a self-care routine to nourish your mental clarity and emotional well-being is essential during this time.

1. Prioritize Sleep

Sleep disruptions, such as night sweats and insomnia, can worsen mood swings and cloud mental clarity. Establishing a healthy sleep routine will help you feel more rested and mentally sharp.

- **Sleep Hygiene Tips:** Stick to a consistent sleep schedule, create a calming bedtime routine, and keep your bedroom cool and dark to minimize night sweats.

- **Relaxation Techniques:** Practices like deep breathing, progressive muscle relaxation, or listening to calming music before bed can help you wind down.

2. Engage in Brain-Boosting Activities

Keeping your brain active can combat menopause-related cognitive changes and improve focus.

- **Mental Stimulation:** Engage in puzzles, reading, writing, or learning new skills to keep your brain sharp. Consider taking up a new hobby that challenges your cognitive abilities, such as learning a language or a musical instrument.

- **Social Connection:** Interacting with others keeps your mind engaged and boosts mental well-being. Make time for meaningful conversations with friends, or join a group or class that interests you.

3. Nourish Your Body and Mind with a Balanced Diet

What you eat can directly affect how you feel mentally and emotionally.

- **Focus on Omega-3s and Antioxidants:** Fatty fish, flaxseeds, walnuts, and leafy greens are rich in omega-3 fatty acids and antioxidants that promote brain health and reduce inflammation.

- **Mindful Eating:** Be present when you eat—enjoy your meals without distractions, and choose foods that make you feel good physically and emotionally.

4. Pamper Yourself

Self-care isn't selfish—it's essential for maintaining mental and emotional balance.

- **Schedule "Me Time":** Whether it's a long bath, a massage, or simply reading a good book, carve out time to do something that brings you joy and relaxation.

- **Daily Gratitude Practice:** Write down a few things you're grateful for each day. Focusing on the positive can improve your emotional outlook and reduce stress.

Mindfulness and Meditation: Techniques for Relaxation

Mindfulness and meditation are powerful tools for calming your mind, reducing stress, and gaining clarity during menopause. These practices help you stay present, manage emotional reactivity, and cultivate inner peace.

1. Mindfulness Meditation

Mindfulness is the practice of being fully present and aware of your thoughts, feelings, and surroundings without judgment. Regular mindfulness meditation can help you manage stress and emotional changes more effectively.

- **How to Practice:** Sit in a quiet space and focus on your breath. If your mind wanders, gently bring your focus back to your breath without criticism. Start with just five minutes a day, gradually increasing as you become more comfortable with the practice.

- **Benefit:** Studies have shown that mindfulness meditation can reduce symptoms of anxiety, depression, and mood swings in menopausal women.

2. Body Scan Meditation

A body scan meditation helps you relax by bringing awareness to each part of your body, releasing tension, and cultivating a sense of calm.

- **How to Practice:** Lie down or sit comfortably. Starting from your toes, mentally "scan" your body, noticing any tension or discomfort. Breathe into each area, consciously relaxing as you move up your body.

- **Benefit:** This practice helps release physical stress, which can lead to mental and emotional relaxation as well.

3. Guided Imagery

Guided imagery involves visualizing a calming place or scenario to help reduce stress and bring about emotional tranquility.

- **How to Practice:** Find a quiet space and close your eyes. Imagine yourself in a peaceful setting—a beach, a forest, or a garden. Focus on the details of this place: the sounds, smells, and sights. Let yourself fully immerse in the relaxation of the scene.

- **Benefit:** Visualization can reduce stress and anxiety, improving your overall emotional resilience.

Redefining Yourself: Embracing the Opportunity for Personal Growth

Menopause is not just an ending; it's the beginning of a new phase in life. While the physical and emotional changes can be challenging, this transition also presents a unique opportunity for self-discovery, reinvention, and personal growth.

1. Letting Go of Old Identities

As menopause marks the end of your reproductive years, it's natural to feel a sense of loss. However, it's also a chance to let go of past roles or expectations that may no longer serve you.

- **Reflection Exercise:** Take time to reflect on the roles you've played throughout your life (mother, partner, professional, caregiver) and ask yourself which roles you want to continue and which you're ready to let go of.

2. Embracing Change as a Time for Growth

Rather than fearing the changes that come with menopause, embrace them as a catalyst for personal growth.

- **Explore New Interests:** Now is the time to pursue passions or hobbies that you may have set aside earlier in life. Whether it's painting, traveling, or starting a new career, menopause can be a period of exciting self-discovery.

- **Challenge Yourself:** Push yourself out of your comfort zone by trying new activities, setting new goals, or engaging in personal development. Growth often comes from stepping into the unfamiliar.

3. Cultivating Self-Compassion

Menopause is a time to be kind to yourself. You're navigating a major life transition, and it's important to give yourself grace as you adjust to the changes.

- **Self-Compassion Practice:** Speak to yourself as you would to a close friend. When you experience difficulties, remind yourself that it's okay to feel vulnerable and that you're doing the best you can.

- **Affirmations:** Use positive affirmations to reinforce self-compassion. Phrases like "I am strong" or "I embrace change with grace" can shift your mindset toward one of growth and positivity.

4. Redefining Your Future

Menopause is a time to reimagine the future and set new intentions for the next phase of your life.

- **Vision Board:** Create a vision board that reflects your goals and aspirations for this next chapter. Whether it's focusing on health, relationships, or personal achievements, visualizing your future can inspire you to take meaningful steps toward those goals.

- **Personal Mission Statement:** Write a personal mission statement that captures who you want to become in this new phase. Use it as a guide for decisions, helping you stay aligned with your values and aspirations.

Menopause is a significant emotional and mental transition, but it's also an invitation to redefine yourself and embrace new possibilities. By managing mood swings, adopting self-care routines, practicing mindfulness, and exploring personal growth, you can turn this phase into an empowering experience. Menopause doesn't have to be a period of loss or confusion—it can be a time of rejuvenation, clarity, and transformation. Take this opportunity to reconnect with yourself, nurture your emotional well-being, and step into this new chapter with confidence and optimism.

Chapter 7

Nourishing Your Body: Food and Nutrition for Midlife

As you navigate the changes of menopause, your dietary choices can play a crucial role in managing symptoms and supporting your overall health. The right nutrition can help balance hormones, boost energy, and maintain the health of your skin, hair, and bones. This chapter explores the menopause diet, highlights superfoods, offers strategies for fighting fatigue, and provides insights into supplements that can enhance your well-being during this transition.

The Menopause Diet: Foods to Help Balance Hormones

Eating a well-balanced diet can help alleviate some of the symptoms associated with menopause. Incorporating hormone-balancing foods can improve mood, reduce hot flashes, and promote overall health.

1. Focus on Phytoestrogens

Phytoestrogens are plant-based compounds that mimic estrogen in the body. They can help balance hormone levels and reduce menopausal symptoms.

- **Sources:** Include foods such as:

  - **Soy Products:** Tofu, tempeh, and edamame are rich in isoflavones, a type of phytoestrogen.

  - **Flaxseeds:** Ground flaxseeds can be added to smoothies, oatmeal, or yogurt for an extra boost.

  - **Legumes:** Chickpeas, lentils, and beans are excellent sources of fiber and phytoestrogens.

2. Incorporate Healthy Fats

Healthy fats are vital for hormone production and overall health. Omega-3 fatty acids, in particular, can help reduce inflammation and improve heart health.

- **Sources:** Opt for:

  - **Fatty Fish:** Salmon, mackerel, and sardines are rich in omega-3s.

  - **Nuts and Seeds:** Walnuts, chia seeds, and flaxseeds provide healthy fats and protein.

  - **Avocado:** A great source of healthy monounsaturated fats, avocados can be enjoyed in salads or on whole-grain toast.

3. Embrace Whole Grains

Whole grains are essential for providing stable energy and important nutrients.

- **Sources:** Choose whole grains like:

  - **Quinoa:** A complete protein that's also high in fiber and minerals.

  - **Brown Rice:** Provides essential nutrients and keeps you feeling full.

  - **Oats:** A great source of soluble fiber that can help manage cholesterol levels.

4. Prioritize Fruits and Vegetables

Fruits and vegetables are packed with vitamins, minerals, and antioxidants that support overall health and well-being.

- **Best Choices:** Focus on:

  - **Berries:** Blueberries, strawberries, and raspberries are rich in antioxidants and can help fight inflammation.

  - **Cruciferous Vegetables:** Broccoli, cauliflower, and Brussels sprouts support liver function and help metabolize hormones.

  - **Leafy Greens:** Spinach, kale, and Swiss chard are high in nutrients and can help combat fatigue.

5. Stay Hydrated

Staying hydrated is crucial for managing symptoms like hot flashes and maintaining overall health.

- **Water Intake:** Aim for at least 8-10 cups of water daily. Herbal teas, coconut water, and clear soups can also help keep you hydrated.

- **Limit Caffeine and Alcohol:** Both can exacerbate hot flashes and disrupt sleep, so moderation is key.

Superfoods for Skin, Hair, and Bone Health

Menopause can impact your skin, hair, and bone density, making it essential to nourish your body with superfoods that support these areas.

1. Skin Health

Hormonal changes during menopause can lead to dryness and loss of elasticity in the skin.

- **Superfoods:**

    - **Avocado:** Rich in healthy fats and vitamins C and E, avocados support skin hydration and elasticity.

    - **Berries:** High in antioxidants, berries help combat oxidative stress, which can age the skin.

    - **Sweet Potatoes:** Packed with beta-carotene, sweet potatoes can help promote skin health and repair.

2. Hair Health

Changes in hormone levels can lead to thinning hair or hair loss.

- **Superfoods:**

    - **Eggs:** A great source of biotin and protein, which are essential for healthy hair growth.

- o **Spinach:** High in iron and vitamins A and C, spinach helps nourish hair follicles.

  - o **Salmon:** Provides omega-3 fatty acids that promote scalp health and shine.

3. Bone Health

Estrogen plays a significant role in maintaining bone density, and its decline during menopause can increase the risk of osteoporosis.

- **Superfoods:**

  - o **Dairy Products:** Milk, yogurt, and cheese are excellent sources of calcium and vitamin D, both essential for bone health.

  - o **Almonds:** High in calcium and magnesium, almonds support bone density.

  - o **Leafy Greens:** Kale, bok choy, and collard greens provide both calcium and vitamin K, which is important for bone health.

Fighting Fatigue and Boosting Energy Naturally

Fatigue is a common complaint during menopause, often exacerbated by sleep disturbances and hormonal changes. Here are strategies to boost your energy levels naturally:

1. Prioritize Quality Sleep

Restorative sleep is essential for maintaining energy levels.

- **Sleep Hygiene Tips:**

  - o Stick to a regular sleep schedule.

  - o Create a calming bedtime routine that includes relaxation techniques such as reading or meditation.

  - o Keep your bedroom dark, quiet, and cool.

2. Choose Energizing Foods

Certain foods can provide lasting energy without causing crashes.

- **Energy-Boosting Options:**

  - **Complex Carbohydrates:** Whole grains, fruits, and vegetables provide steady energy.

  - **Lean Proteins:** Chicken, turkey, tofu, and legumes support sustained energy levels and muscle maintenance.

  - **Nuts and Seeds:** A handful of almonds or walnuts can provide a quick energy boost.

3. Stay Active

Regular physical activity is a natural way to increase energy levels.

- **Exercise Recommendations:**

  - Aim for at least 150 minutes of moderate aerobic exercise per week, such as brisk walking, swimming, or cycling.

  - Include strength training exercises twice a week to build muscle mass and boost metabolism.

4. Manage Stress

Chronic stress can lead to fatigue and burnout.

- **Stress-Relief Techniques:**

  - Engage in relaxation practices like yoga, meditation, or deep-breathing exercises.

  - Spend time in nature or practice hobbies that bring you joy to recharge your mental energy.

Supplements: Which Ones Help and Which to Avoid

While a balanced diet should provide most of the nutrients you need, certain supplements can support your health during menopause. However, it's essential to choose wisely.

1. Beneficial Supplements

- **Calcium and Vitamin D:** Essential for maintaining bone density. Aim for 1,200 mg of calcium and 800-1,000 IU of vitamin D daily, especially if you have limited sun exposure.

- **Omega-3 Fatty Acids:** Fish oil supplements can help reduce inflammation, improve heart health, and potentially alleviate mood swings.

- **Magnesium:** Supports muscle and nerve function and can help with sleep. The recommended daily allowance is around 320 mg for women.

- **Vitamin E:** May help alleviate hot flashes and improve skin health. A dose of 400 IU daily is generally considered safe.

2. Supplements to Avoid

- **Unregulated Herbal Supplements:** While some herbal remedies may help with symptoms, many lack regulation and can interact with medications. Always consult your healthcare provider before starting any new supplements.

- **Excessive Iron:** Unless diagnosed with iron deficiency, avoid iron supplements, as excess iron can be harmful.

- **High-Dose Supplements:** Large doses of any vitamin or mineral can lead to toxicity. Stick to the recommended daily allowances unless otherwise directed by a healthcare professional.

Nourishing your body with the right foods and supplements during menopause can significantly impact your health and well-being. By embracing a hormone-balancing diet, incorporating superfoods, addressing fatigue naturally, and carefully selecting supplements, you can support your body through this transition. Remember, this is a time for self-care and nurturing your health, so take the time to explore new recipes, experiment with different foods, and find what works best for you. Your body deserves it, and you'll emerge from this chapter feeling stronger and more vibrant than ever.

Chapter 8

Fitness at Any Age: Moving Your Body Through Menopause

Staying active during menopause is essential for maintaining physical health, mental clarity, and emotional well-being. Regular exercise can help alleviate common symptoms, enhance bone health, and improve overall quality of life. This chapter will explore the importance of strength training, low-impact exercises, the benefits of yoga and Pilates, and strategies to stay motivated and make fitness an enjoyable part of your daily routine.

Strength Training and Bone Health: Why Muscle Matters

As estrogen levels decline during menopause, women may experience a decrease in bone density, increasing the risk of osteoporosis. Strength training is one of the most effective ways to combat this and improve overall health.

1. The Importance of Muscle Mass

- **Increased Metabolism:** Muscle tissue burns more calories at rest than fat tissue, helping to maintain a healthy weight.

- **Bone Density:** Strength training stimulates bone growth and can help prevent bone loss. The mechanical stress placed on bones during resistance training promotes bone density and strength.

- **Functional Strength:** Building muscle improves your ability to perform daily activities, reducing the risk of falls and injuries.

2. Types of Strength Training

- **Weight Lifting:** Using free weights or machines can effectively build strength. Start with lighter weights and gradually increase as you gain confidence and strength.

- **Bodyweight Exercises:** Exercises like squats, lunges, and push-ups use your own body weight to build muscle and can be done anywhere.

- **Resistance Bands:** These portable bands provide resistance during exercises and are excellent for both beginners and advanced fitness enthusiasts.

3. Creating a Strength Training Routine

- **Frequency:** Aim for at least two to three days a week of strength training, allowing for rest days in between.

- **Repetitions and Sets:** Start with 1-2 sets of 10-15 repetitions for each exercise, focusing on proper form over heavy weights.

- **Target Major Muscle Groups:** Include exercises that target all major muscle groups, such as legs, back, chest, and core.

Low-Impact Exercises for Joint Health and Flexibility

Menopause can sometimes bring joint pain or stiffness, making low-impact exercises essential for maintaining mobility and flexibility without adding strain to the joints.

1. Benefits of Low-Impact Exercise

- **Joint-Friendly:** Low-impact exercises reduce the stress on joints while still providing cardiovascular benefits and improving overall fitness.

- **Reduced Injury Risk:** These exercises are generally safer and less likely to lead to injuries compared to high-impact activities.

2. Recommended Low-Impact Exercises

- **Walking:** A simple and accessible way to stay active. Aim for brisk walks to elevate your heart rate while being gentle on your joints.

- **Swimming:** Offers a full-body workout with minimal impact on joints. The buoyancy of water reduces stress while providing resistance.

- **Cycling:** Whether on a stationary bike or cycling outdoors, this activity improves cardiovascular fitness and builds leg strength without impacting your joints.

- **Elliptical Machines:** These machines mimic the motion of running without the impact, providing a great cardiovascular workout.

3. Flexibility and Mobility Exercises

- **Stretching:** Incorporate stretching into your routine to maintain flexibility and prevent stiffness. Focus on major muscle groups and hold stretches for 15-30 seconds.

- **Foam Rolling:** This technique helps relieve muscle tightness and improve flexibility by rolling out sore spots.

The Role of Yoga and Pilates in Easing Symptoms

Yoga and Pilates are excellent complementary forms of exercise during menopause. They enhance flexibility, strength, and mental well-being while providing relief from common menopausal symptoms.

1. Yoga Benefits

- **Stress Reduction:** Yoga emphasizes mindfulness and deep breathing, which can help manage stress and anxiety associated with menopause.

- **Improved Sleep:** Regular practice can enhance sleep quality and help combat insomnia, a common symptom during menopause.

- **Relief from Hot Flashes:** Some studies suggest that yoga may help reduce the frequency and intensity of hot flashes.

2. Pilates Benefits

- **Core Strengthening:** Pilates focuses on core stability, which supports posture and overall strength. A strong core can help prevent back pain, which can be common during menopause.

- **Improved Flexibility and Balance:** The controlled movements in Pilates enhance flexibility and balance, reducing the risk of falls.

3. Incorporating Yoga and Pilates

- **Classes and Online Resources:** Many gyms, community centers, and online platforms offer yoga and Pilates classes tailored for various fitness levels.

- **Home Practice:** Consider following online videos or apps that guide you through routines at home. Even a short 10-15 minute practice can be beneficial.

How to Stay Motivated and Make Exercise Enjoyable

Finding the motivation to exercise regularly can be challenging, especially during menopause when energy levels may fluctuate. However, incorporating enjoyable activities and setting realistic goals can help keep you engaged and committed to your fitness journey.

1. Set Realistic Goals

- **SMART Goals:** Use the SMART framework—Specific, Measurable, Achievable, Relevant, and Time-bound—to set your fitness goals. For example, aim to walk 30 minutes three times a week for the next month.

- **Celebrate Small Wins:** Acknowledge and celebrate your progress, whether it's completing a workout, lifting heavier weights, or simply feeling more energetic.

2. Find Activities You Enjoy

- **Explore Different Options:** Try various fitness classes, outdoor activities, or sports to find what you love. Experiment with dancing, hiking, or group fitness classes to keep things fresh.

- **Mix It Up:** Combine different types of exercise—strength training, cardio, yoga, and fun activities—to prevent boredom and keep your routine dynamic.

3. Make Exercise a Social Activity

- **Work Out with Friends:** Join a friend for workouts or classes. Exercising with others can boost motivation and make fitness more enjoyable.

- **Join a Group:** Look for local fitness groups, clubs, or classes that align with your interests. The camaraderie can provide accountability and support.

4. Listen to Your Body

- **Pay Attention to Your Needs:** During menopause, it's important to listen to your body and adjust your exercise routine as needed. If you're feeling fatigued, opt for a gentler workout.

- **Rest and Recovery:** Don't forget to allow for rest days to help your body recover and prevent burnout.

Staying physically active during menopause is crucial for maintaining overall health, enhancing mood, and alleviating common symptoms. By incorporating strength training, low-impact exercises, yoga, and Pilates into your routine, you can support your body through this transitional phase of life. Remember that fitness should be enjoyable and tailored to your unique needs, so find activities that resonate with you and celebrate your progress along the way. With commitment and positivity, you can thrive during menopause and embrace a healthier, more vibrant life.

Chapter 9

Sleep Solutions: How to Rest Easy

Menopause often brings sleep disruptions, including insomnia, night sweats, and hot flashes, making restful sleep more elusive. Yet, good quality sleep is essential for hormonal balance, emotional well-being, and overall health. In this chapter, we'll explore effective strategies for establishing a bedtime routine, herbal remedies, techniques to combat night sweats, and the crucial role of sleep in hormonal health.

Building a Bedtime Routine that Works

Creating a calming bedtime routine can signal to your body that it's time to wind down and prepare for restful sleep.

1. Consistency is Key

- **Set a Schedule:** Aim to go to bed and wake up at the same time each day, even on weekends. This helps regulate your body's internal clock.

- **Wind Down Period:** Start your bedtime routine 30-60 minutes before sleep. Engage in calming activities that promote relaxation.

2. Create a Calming Environment

- **Bedroom Setup:** Make your bedroom a sleep sanctuary by keeping it cool, dark, and quiet. Consider using blackout curtains and a white noise machine or earplugs if necessary.

- **Comfortable Bedding:** Invest in a comfortable mattress and pillows that suit your sleeping position. The right bedding can significantly enhance sleep quality.

3. Relaxation Techniques

- **Mindful Breathing:** Practice deep breathing exercises or progressive muscle relaxation to calm your mind and body before bed.

- **Gentle Stretching:** Incorporate light stretches or yoga poses to relieve tension and prepare your body for sleep.

4. Limit Stimulants

- **Avoid Screens:** Reduce exposure to screens (TV, smartphones, tablets) at least an hour before bed. The blue light emitted can interfere with melatonin production, disrupting sleep.

- **Watch Your Diet:** Limit caffeine and nicotine in the afternoon and evening, as both can interfere with your ability to fall asleep.

Herbal Remedies and Natural Sleep Aids

Several herbal remedies and natural sleep aids can promote relaxation and improve sleep quality during menopause.

1. Valerian Root

- **Benefits:** Valerian root is a popular herbal remedy known for its sedative properties. It may help reduce the time it takes to fall asleep and improve sleep quality.

- **Usage:** Available in tea, capsules, or tinctures. Consult your healthcare provider for appropriate dosages.

2. Chamomile

- **Benefits:** Chamomile tea is often used for its calming effects and can help reduce anxiety and promote sleep.

- **Usage:** Drink a cup of chamomile tea 30 minutes before bedtime for optimal results.

3. Lavender

- **Benefits:** Lavender is known for its relaxing aroma and can help reduce anxiety and improve sleep quality.

- **Usage:** Consider using lavender essential oil in a diffuser, adding it to a warm bath, or using lavender sachets in your pillow.

4. Melatonin

- **Benefits:** Melatonin is a hormone that regulates sleep-wake cycles. Supplementation can be beneficial for some women experiencing insomnia during menopause.

- **Usage:** Take melatonin supplements 30-60 minutes before bedtime. Consult with your healthcare provider for the right dosage.

Overcoming Night Sweats and Hot Flashes at Night

Night sweats and hot flashes can significantly disrupt sleep, but several strategies can help you manage these symptoms effectively.

1. Keep Cool

- **Temperature Control:** Keep your bedroom cool (around 60-67°F or 15-19°C) to help reduce the likelihood of night sweats. Use fans, air conditioning, or open windows to circulate air.

- **Cooling Bedding:** Invest in moisture-wicking sheets and lightweight blankets designed to keep you cool throughout the night.

2. Layer Your Bedding

- **Use Layers:** Dress in lightweight, breathable fabrics and use layers for your bedding so you can easily adjust if you feel too hot or too cold during the night.

3. Hydration and Diet

- **Stay Hydrated:** Drink plenty of water throughout the day, but limit fluids right before bedtime to minimize nighttime bathroom trips.

- **Avoid Triggers:** Identify and avoid foods or drinks that may trigger hot flashes, such as spicy foods, caffeine, and alcohol.

4. Practice Relaxation Techniques

- **Cool Down Before Bed:** Engage in relaxing activities such as a warm bath or meditation before bed to help calm your body and mind.

- **Cooling Products:** Consider using cooling pillows or gel-infused mattress toppers to provide additional relief from night sweats.

The Importance of Rest for Hormonal Balance

Rest is vital for hormonal balance and overall health, especially during menopause.

1. Hormonal Regulation

- **Impact on Hormones:** Lack of sleep can disrupt the balance of hormones like cortisol, insulin, and growth hormone, potentially worsening menopausal symptoms.

- **Stress Management:** Adequate sleep helps manage stress levels, which can positively influence hormonal health.

2. Mood and Cognitive Function

- **Mental Health:** Quality sleep supports emotional well-being and cognitive function. Poor sleep can lead to irritability, anxiety, and difficulty concentrating, which can be exacerbated during menopause.

- **Memory and Focus:** Good sleep enhances memory consolidation and cognitive performance, helping you stay sharp and focused.

3. Physical Health

- **Immune Function:** Sleep plays a crucial role in supporting a healthy immune system, helping your body fend off illness and infection.

- **Weight Management:** Restful sleep can influence weight regulation by supporting healthy metabolism and reducing cravings for unhealthy foods.

Getting quality sleep during menopause can be challenging, but it's vital for maintaining hormonal balance and overall health. By establishing a calming bedtime routine, exploring herbal remedies, managing night sweats, and prioritizing rest, you can significantly improve your sleep quality. Remember, you're not alone in this journey, and seeking support from healthcare professionals and loved ones can further enhance your ability to embrace this transition with confidence and grace. As you nurture your body with restorative sleep, you'll find the strength to thrive in this new chapter of life.

Chapter 10

Rekindling Your Relationships and Sex Life

Menopause can usher in significant changes to your sexual health and relationships. While this transition may bring challenges, it can also be an opportunity to deepen intimacy and reconnect with your partner. In this chapter, we'll explore how menopause affects libido, the importance of open communication, strategies for managing vaginal health, and ways to rediscover passion in your relationship.

The Intimacy Shift: How Menopause Affects Your Libido

The hormonal fluctuations associated with menopause can lead to changes in sexual desire, making it crucial to understand how these shifts may impact your intimacy.

1. Hormonal Changes and Libido

- **Estrogen Decline:** As estrogen levels drop, you may experience a decrease in libido. This can manifest as a reduced interest in sex or difficulty becoming aroused.

- **Testosterone Levels:** While testosterone is often considered a male hormone, women also produce it, and levels can fluctuate during menopause. This fluctuation can affect sexual desire and pleasure.

2. Emotional and Psychological Factors

- **Body Image:** Many women experience changes in body shape and weight during menopause, which can impact self-esteem and confidence, leading to decreased sexual desire.

- **Mood Changes:** Mood swings, anxiety, and depression associated with menopause can also contribute to reduced libido.

3. Normalizing the Change

- **Understanding the Shift:** Recognize that changes in libido are a common experience during menopause and that it's important to approach these changes with patience and understanding.

- **Explore New Forms of Intimacy:** Intimacy is not solely about sexual activity. Explore other ways to connect with your partner, such as cuddling, holding hands, or engaging in shared activities.

Open Communication with Your Partner: Talking About Changes

Communication is vital for navigating the changes that menopause brings to your relationship and sex life.

1. Create a Safe Space for Dialogue

- **Choose the Right Time:** Initiate conversations about sexual health and intimacy in a comfortable setting where both partners feel relaxed and free to express themselves.

- **Be Honest and Open:** Share your feelings, concerns, and experiences related to menopause and intimacy. Honesty fosters understanding and support between partners.

2. Discuss Changes Together

- **Explore Each Other's Needs:** Encourage your partner to share their thoughts and feelings about the changes you're both experiencing. This can help you both understand each other's needs better.

- **Reassure Each Other:** Discuss the importance of your relationship and reassure each other that intimacy can be redefined during this transition.

3. Seek Professional Guidance

- **Therapy or Counseling:** Consider seeking the help of a therapist or counselor specializing in sexual health and relationships. Professional guidance can provide additional strategies for navigating these changes together.

Vaginal Health: Combating Dryness, Discomfort, and Pain

Vaginal dryness and discomfort are common issues that many women experience during menopause, but there are effective solutions to enhance vaginal health.

1. Understanding Vaginal Dryness

- **Hormonal Changes:** As estrogen levels decline, vaginal tissues can become thinner, drier, and less elastic, leading to discomfort during sex.

- **Impact on Intimacy:** Vaginal dryness can affect sexual pleasure and lead to a decrease in libido, creating a cycle of frustration and avoidance.

2. Effective Solutions

- **Water-Based Lubricants:** Using a water-based lubricant during intercourse can help alleviate dryness and enhance comfort. Avoid products with irritating ingredients such as glycerin or fragrances.

- **Vaginal Moisturizers:** Over-the-counter vaginal moisturizers can help maintain vaginal moisture and improve comfort during daily activities and intercourse.

- **Prescription Options:** Consult your healthcare provider about hormone therapy options or other medications that can help alleviate symptoms of vaginal dryness.

3. Pelvic Floor Exercises

- **Kegel Exercises:** Strengthening the pelvic floor muscles can improve vaginal tone and enhance sexual sensation. Practice Kegel exercises by contracting and relaxing the pelvic muscles.

- **Physical Therapy:** A pelvic floor physical therapist can provide personalized exercises and techniques to strengthen pelvic muscles and improve sexual function.

Rediscovering Passion: Sex After Menopause

Menopause doesn't have to mean the end of a satisfying sex life. Instead, it can be a chance to explore new dimensions of intimacy and pleasure.

1. Explore New Avenues of Pleasure

- **Experimentation:** Embrace this time as an opportunity to explore new sexual experiences, positions, or fantasies. Openly discussing desires can enhance intimacy.

- **Sensual Activities:** Engage in activities that promote sensuality, such as massages, bubble baths, or shared experiences that encourage closeness and intimacy.

2. Focus on Foreplay

- **Prioritize Foreplay:** Spending more time on foreplay can enhance arousal and make sex more enjoyable. Experiment with different types of foreplay, such as kissing, touching, or oral stimulation.

- **Incorporate Intimacy Practices:** Consider adding intimacy practices such as tantra, which emphasizes connection and mindfulness during sexual experiences.

3. Adjust Expectations

- **Shift Your Mindset:** Embrace the idea that intimacy can change over time and that it's okay to redefine what a satisfying sex life looks like for you and your partner.

- **Create an Intimate Atmosphere:** Setting the mood with candles, music, or other sensual elements can enhance the experience and promote a sense of connection.

Menopause is a significant transition that can impact various aspects of your relationships and sexual health. By understanding the intimacy shift, fostering open communication, addressing vaginal health concerns, and rediscovering passion, you can navigate this journey with confidence and grace. Embrace this chapter as an opportunity for growth and connection, recognizing that intimacy can evolve and deepen in new and fulfilling ways. With patience and mutual support, you can continue to nurture your relationship and enjoy a vibrant and satisfying sex life beyond menopause.

Chapter 11

Skin Deep: Taking Care of Your Skin, Hair, and Nails

As women transition through menopause, they often experience various changes in their skin, hair, and nails due to hormonal fluctuations. These changes can affect confidence and self-esteem, but with the right knowledge and care strategies, you can maintain your radiance. In this chapter, we will explore why these changes happen, provide anti-aging tips, address hair thinning and loss, and offer self-care rituals to boost confidence and enhance your natural beauty.

Why Skin Changes Happen and What You Can Do

The hormonal changes during menopause significantly impact the skin, often leading to dryness, loss of elasticity, and changes in texture.

1. The Role of Hormones

- **Decline in Estrogen:** The decrease in estrogen levels during menopause can lead to reduced collagen production, which is crucial for maintaining skin elasticity and firmness.

- **Impact on Moisture Levels:** Lower estrogen can also reduce the skin's ability to retain moisture, leading to dryness and increased sensitivity.

2. Common Skin Changes

- **Dryness:** Women may notice their skin becoming drier and less supple, leading to itchiness and irritation.

- **Wrinkles and Fine Lines:** The skin may start showing more visible signs of aging, such as wrinkles and fine lines, particularly around the eyes and mouth.

- **Age Spots:** Hyperpigmentation, or age spots, can become more prominent due to prolonged sun exposure and hormonal changes.

3. What You Can Do

- **Hydration:** Drink plenty of water to help maintain skin hydration from the inside out.

- **Moisturizers:** Use rich, hydrating moisturizers that contain ingredients like hyaluronic acid, glycerin, and ceramides to help lock in moisture.

- **Sun Protection:** Apply a broad-spectrum sunscreen with an SPF of at least 30 daily to protect against UV damage, which can exacerbate skin aging.

Anti-Aging Tips: From Moisturizers to Serums

A well-curated skincare routine can help combat the signs of aging and promote a healthy, youthful glow.

1. Building a Skincare Routine

- **Cleanser:** Start with a gentle, hydrating cleanser that won't strip your skin of its natural oils.

- **Toner:** Use an alcohol-free toner to balance the skin's pH and prepare it for further treatments.

2. Key Ingredients to Look For

- **Retinol:** Retinol is a potent ingredient that can help stimulate collagen production, reduce the appearance of fine lines, and improve skin texture.

- **Antioxidants:** Look for serums containing antioxidants like vitamin C, which can help brighten the skin and protect against free radical damage.

- **Peptides:** These can support collagen production and improve skin elasticity.

3. Moisturizers and Hydrating Treatments

- **Heavy Creams:** As skin becomes drier, consider richer creams or oil-based moisturizers in the evening to help seal in moisture overnight.

- **Facial Oils:** Incorporating facial oils can provide additional hydration and nourishment, particularly for dry patches.

4. Regular Exfoliation

- **Chemical Exfoliants:** Use exfoliants containing alpha hydroxy acids (AHAs) or beta hydroxy acids (BHAs) to gently remove dead skin cells and promote cell turnover.

- **Frequency:** Aim to exfoliate 1-2 times per week, adjusting based on your skin's sensitivity.

Dealing with Hair Thinning and Loss

Many women notice changes in their hair, including thinning and increased hair loss, during menopause. Understanding the causes and exploring solutions can help manage these concerns.

1. Causes of Hair Changes

- **Hormonal Fluctuations:** The decline in estrogen and progesterone can lead to hair thinning, as these hormones play a role in hair growth cycles.

- **Dihydrotestosterone (DHT):** An increase in the hormone DHT can contribute to hair loss, particularly in genetically predisposed women.

2. Solutions for Thinning Hair

- **Hair Care Products:** Look for shampoos and conditioners specifically formulated to add volume and promote hair health. Products with biotin and other vitamins can be beneficial.

- **Scalp Treatments:** Consider scalp treatments that stimulate blood circulation and promote hair growth. Ingredients like caffeine and peppermint oil may help invigorate the scalp.

3. Dietary Considerations

- **Nutrition:** Ensure you're getting enough protein, iron, and essential fatty acids in your diet to support hair health. Foods rich in omega-3 fatty acids (such as salmon and walnuts) and antioxidants (like berries) are particularly beneficial.

- **Supplements:** Talk to your healthcare provider about supplements such as biotin, vitamin D, and iron if you suspect nutrient deficiencies.

4. Professional Help

- **Dermatologist Consultation:** If hair thinning is significant, consult a dermatologist for tailored advice and potential treatments, such as topical minoxidil.

Self-Care Rituals for Confidence and Radiance

Self-care is essential for boosting confidence and embracing your beauty during menopause. Incorporating rituals that prioritize your physical and emotional well-being can significantly enhance your overall radiance.

1. Pamper Yourself

- **Spa Days at Home:** Treat yourself to at-home spa days with facials, hair masks, and relaxing baths. Use products that nourish your skin and hair to feel rejuvenated.

- **Mindfulness Practices:** Incorporate mindfulness practices like meditation or yoga to reduce stress and enhance mental clarity.

2. Dress for Confidence

- **Wardrobe Refresh:** Update your wardrobe with flattering clothing that makes you feel confident. Choose fabrics and colors that enhance your features and reflect your personality.

- **Grooming Habits:** Regular grooming, such as manicures and pedicures, can boost confidence and self-esteem. Prioritize self-care as an essential part of your routine.

3. Connect with Others

- **Support Networks:** Engage with friends or support groups to share experiences and tips. Connection with others can provide emotional support and enhance feelings of community.

- **Share Your Journey:** Consider documenting your menopause journey, whether through writing, art, or blogging, to empower yourself and connect with others.

4. Celebrate Your Beauty

- **Affirmations:** Use positive affirmations to reinforce self-love and acceptance. Acknowledge your unique beauty and the wisdom that comes with age.

- **Daily Rituals:** Incorporate small daily rituals that celebrate your body, such as practicing gratitude or appreciating your skin and hair.

Taking care of your skin, hair, and nails during menopause is crucial for maintaining your confidence and sense of self. By understanding the changes that occur, implementing effective skincare and hair care routines, and embracing self-care rituals, you can enhance your natural beauty and radiance. Remember that this phase of life is not just about dealing with challenges but also about celebrating the wisdom, strength, and beauty that come with it. Embrace the journey with self-love, patience, and the knowledge that you can continue to shine brightly at every stage of life.

Chapter 12

Holistic Healing: Alternative Therapies for Menopause Relief

As women navigate the challenges of menopause, many seek alternative therapies to complement traditional medical approaches. Holistic healing focuses on the whole person—mind, body, and spirit—offering various strategies to alleviate symptoms and promote overall well-being. In this chapter, we will explore the benefits of acupuncture, reflexology, and massage, discuss herbal remedies, delve into aromatherapy and essential oils, and highlight the importance of finding the right combination of Eastern and Western approaches that work for you.

Acupuncture, Reflexology, and Massage: How They Help

Alternative therapies such as acupuncture, reflexology, and massage can provide significant relief from menopause symptoms by addressing both physical and emotional issues.

1. Acupuncture

- **What It Is:** Acupuncture is a traditional Chinese medicine practice that involves inserting thin needles into specific points on the body to balance energy (or "qi") and promote healing.

- **Benefits for Menopause:**

  - **Hot Flashes:** Research suggests that acupuncture may reduce the frequency and intensity of hot flashes.

  - **Mood Regulation:** It can help alleviate anxiety and improve mood, making it easier to cope with emotional changes during menopause.

  - **Sleep Improvement:** Acupuncture may improve sleep quality, addressing insomnia often associated with menopause.

2. Reflexology

- **What It Is:** Reflexology is a therapeutic practice that involves applying pressure to specific points on the feet, hands, or ears that correspond to different body organs and systems.

- **Benefits for Menopause:**

  - **Stress Relief:** Reflexology promotes relaxation and reduces stress, which can be particularly beneficial for managing mood swings and emotional health.

  - **Hormonal Balance:** It may support hormonal balance by stimulating endocrine glands, potentially alleviating symptoms like hot flashes and mood changes.

3. Massage

- **What It Is:** Massage therapy involves manipulating the body's soft tissues to promote relaxation, relieve tension, and improve circulation.

- **Benefits for Menopause:**

  - **Physical Relief:** Massage can ease muscle tension and pain, helping to combat physical discomfort associated with menopause.

  - **Emotional Well-Being:** The soothing nature of massage promotes relaxation and can help reduce anxiety, contributing to better emotional health.

Herbal Remedies: From Black Cohosh to Red Clover

Herbal remedies have been used for centuries to alleviate various symptoms associated with menopause. While they can be effective, it's essential to consult with a healthcare professional before starting any herbal treatment.

1. Black Cohosh

- **Overview:** Black cohosh is a plant native to North America often used to treat menopausal symptoms.

- **Benefits:**

    - **Hot Flashes:** Studies suggest that black cohosh may help reduce the frequency and severity of hot flashes.

    - **Mood Improvement:** It may also help improve mood and reduce anxiety in some women.

2. Red Clover

- **Overview:** Red clover is rich in phytoestrogens, plant-derived compounds that mimic estrogen in the body.

- **Benefits:**

    - **Symptom Relief:** It has been found to help reduce hot flashes and improve overall menopausal symptoms.

    - **Bone Health:** Some research indicates that red clover may support bone health, potentially countering menopause-related bone density loss.

3. Other Herbal Options

- **Dong Quai:** Traditionally used in Chinese medicine, Dong Quai may help balance hormones and reduce menopausal symptoms.

- **Evening Primrose Oil:** Often used for breast pain and menopausal symptoms, it may help with hot flashes and mood changes.

Aromatherapy and Essential Oils for Mood and Symptom Management

Aromatherapy utilizes essential oils from plants to promote physical and emotional well-being. Many women find that specific essential oils can help alleviate menopause symptoms.

1. Essential Oils for Hot Flashes

- **Clary Sage:** Known for its calming properties, clary sage can help balance hormones and reduce hot flashes.

- **Peppermint:** This oil can provide a cooling sensation, which may help alleviate the discomfort of hot flashes.

2. Essential Oils for Mood Enhancement

- **Lavender:** Renowned for its calming effects, lavender oil can help reduce anxiety and promote better sleep.

- **Bergamot:** This uplifting oil can improve mood and alleviate stress, making it beneficial for emotional well-being during menopause.

3. Methods of Use

- **Diffusion:** Use a diffuser to disperse essential oils into the air for inhalation.

- **Topical Application:** Dilute essential oils with a carrier oil (like coconut or almond oil) and apply to pulse points for direct benefits.

- **Bathing:** Add a few drops of essential oils to bathwater for a relaxing soak.

Finding What Works for You: Combining Eastern and Western Approaches

Menopause is a unique journey for every woman, and finding the right combination of therapies can enhance your quality of life during this transition.

1. Individualized Approach

- **Trial and Error:** Be open to experimenting with different therapies and remedies to discover what works best for your body and mind.

- **Keep a Journal:** Document your experiences with various treatments, noting what alleviates symptoms and what does not.

2. Integrative Health Care

- **Collaborative Care:** Work with a healthcare provider familiar with both Western and Eastern medicine to create a comprehensive treatment plan tailored to your needs.

- **Holistic Wellness:** Consider therapies that address not just physical symptoms but also emotional and mental well-being, fostering a more holistic approach to health.

3. Community and Support

- **Support Groups:** Engaging with others experiencing similar challenges can provide valuable insights, shared experiences, and emotional support.

- **Professional Guidance:** Seek professionals skilled in integrative medicine, acupuncture, or herbal remedies to help guide your holistic journey through menopause.

Holistic healing offers various alternative therapies that can complement traditional menopause treatments, promoting physical and emotional well-being. By exploring options like acupuncture, reflexology, and massage, as well as herbal remedies and aromatherapy, you can find effective strategies for managing symptoms. Remember, every woman's experience with menopause is unique, so it's essential to find what works best for you. Embrace the journey of discovery, and empower yourself with the knowledge that you have the tools to thrive during this transformative phase of life.

Chapter 13

Life After Menopause: What's Next?

Menopause marks a significant transition in a woman's life, but it is not the end; rather, it is a new beginning filled with opportunities for growth, self-discovery, and revitalization. In this chapter, we will explore what to expect in the postmenopausal phase, how to maintain health and vitality in your later years, strategies for managing osteoporosis and heart health, and how to embrace the chance to reinvent yourself with new goals, hobbies, and passions.

Postmenopause: What to Expect in the Long Term

The postmenopausal phase can bring significant changes, both physically and emotionally. Understanding these changes can help you navigate this new chapter with confidence and resilience.

1. Hormonal Changes

- **Decreased Hormone Levels:** After menopause, estrogen and progesterone levels significantly decline, leading to various changes in the body. This can affect everything from metabolism to mood.

- **Symptom Persistence:** Some women may continue to experience symptoms from the menopausal transition, such as hot flashes or mood swings, though they often become less severe over time.

2. Changes in Menstrual Cycle

- **No Periods:** By definition, a woman is considered postmenopausal when she has not had a menstrual period for 12 consecutive months. The cessation of menstruation marks a significant shift in reproductive health.

3. Long-Term Effects of Menopause

- **Physical Changes:** Expect changes such as weight redistribution, skin changes (like increased dryness), and potential hair thinning. These are normal and can be managed with appropriate self-care.

- **Mental Health:** Some women may experience feelings of loss or identity crisis after menopause. Understanding that this is a natural reaction can help in processing these feelings.

Maintaining Health and Vitality in Your Later Years

Prioritizing health and well-being during the postmenopausal years is essential for maintaining vitality and quality of life.

1. Nutrition and Diet

- **Balanced Diet:** Focus on a diet rich in fruits, vegetables, whole grains, lean proteins, and healthy fats. This can help manage weight, reduce the risk of chronic diseases, and improve overall health.

- **Calcium and Vitamin D:** Ensure adequate intake of calcium and vitamin D to support bone health. Foods rich in calcium include dairy products, leafy greens, and fortified foods. Sun exposure and supplements can provide vitamin D.

2. Regular Exercise

- **Physical Activity:** Engage in regular physical activity that includes cardiovascular, strength training, and flexibility exercises. Aim for at least 150 minutes of moderate aerobic activity per week.

- **Strength Training:** Incorporate strength training at least twice a week to help build muscle mass and bone density, which is crucial in combating osteoporosis.

3. Mental Well-Being

- **Cognitive Health:** Stay mentally active through reading, puzzles, or learning new skills. Activities that challenge your brain can help maintain cognitive function.

- **Stress Management:** Practice stress-reduction techniques such as mindfulness, meditation, or yoga. These practices can promote emotional well-being and resilience.

Managing Osteoporosis and Heart Health

With menopause, the risk for osteoporosis and heart disease increases, making it essential to take proactive steps to manage these health concerns.

1. Understanding Osteoporosis

- **Bone Density Loss:** After menopause, women can lose up to 20% of their bone mass in the first five to seven years. This makes regular bone density screenings essential.

- **Risk Factors:** Other risk factors include family history, low body weight, smoking, excessive alcohol intake, and sedentary lifestyle.

2. Prevention and Management

- **Bone Health Strategies:**

  - **Calcium-Rich Foods:** Incorporate foods high in calcium such as yogurt, cheese, almonds, and dark leafy greens.

  - **Vitamin D:** Ensure sufficient vitamin D intake through diet and sunlight exposure to aid calcium absorption.

  - **Exercise:** Weight-bearing exercises, such as walking, jogging, or dancing, help strengthen bones.

- **Medical Guidance:** Discuss with your healthcare provider the possibility of medications or supplements if you have been diagnosed with osteoporosis.

3. Heart Health Awareness

- **Cardiovascular Risk:** Postmenopausal women are at a higher risk of heart disease due to decreased estrogen levels, which previously offered some protective benefits.

- **Heart Health Strategies:**

  - **Healthy Diet:** Focus on a heart-healthy diet that is low in saturated fats, trans fats, and cholesterol. Emphasize whole grains, fruits, vegetables, and lean proteins.

  - **Regular Check-Ups:** Monitor blood pressure, cholesterol levels, and heart health through regular check-ups with your healthcare provider.

Reinventing Yourself: New Goals, Hobbies, and Passions

The postmenopausal years offer a unique opportunity to redefine yourself, pursue new passions, and set meaningful goals.

1. Embrace New Interests

- **Hobbies:** Explore new hobbies or interests that you may not have had time for previously. This could include painting, gardening, cooking, or learning a musical instrument.

- **Travel and Adventure:** Consider taking up travel, whether local or international, to discover new cultures and experiences. Traveling can be invigorating and provide fresh perspectives.

2. Educational Pursuits

- **Lifelong Learning:** Engage in lifelong learning through courses, workshops, or online classes. This can be a fulfilling way to expand your knowledge and skills.

- **Volunteering:** Get involved in volunteer opportunities within your community. This not only contributes to your community but also offers social connections and a sense of purpose.

3. Setting Goals

- **Personal Goals:** Reflect on personal goals you want to achieve in this new chapter. Consider areas of your life where you'd like to grow, whether it's personal development, fitness, or community engagement.

- **Professional Aspirations:** If you're looking to continue working or start a new career, set professional goals that align with your passions and skills.

Life after menopause is a time of transformation and possibility. By understanding what to expect in the long term, maintaining your health and vitality, managing specific health concerns like osteoporosis and heart health, and embracing new interests and goals, you can thrive beyond menopause. This chapter of life is an opportunity to rediscover yourself, explore new passions, and celebrate the wisdom and experience you have gained. Embrace this journey with confidence, knowing that it's not the end, but a new beginning filled with endless possibilities.

Chapter 14

Building Your Support System

Navigating menopause can feel isolating, but building a strong support system is crucial for thriving during this transition. Whether it's connecting with friends, family, or other women who understand what you're going through, a solid support network can provide valuable insight, encouragement, and companionship. In this chapter, we will explore how to find your tribe, communicate effectively about menopause, navigate challenges in the workplace, and create a menopause-friendly community.

Finding Your Tribe: Connecting with Other Women

Finding a group of like-minded women who understand and share your experiences can be empowering. Here are some ways to connect with others:

1. Local Support Groups

- **Join a Group:** Many communities have support groups specifically for women experiencing menopause. Check local health organizations, community centers, or hospitals for offerings.

- **Online Forums:** Explore online forums and social media groups dedicated to menopause discussions. These platforms allow you to connect with women globally and share experiences and advice.

2. Workshops and Classes

- **Educational Events:** Attend workshops, seminars, or classes focused on menopause and women's health. These events often provide a space for discussion and connection with others facing similar challenges.

- **Fitness or Wellness Classes:** Join fitness or wellness classes that focus on women's health. Participating in these activities can lead to friendships with others who understand your journey.

3. Women's Clubs and Organizations

- **Community Organizations:** Many communities have women's clubs that focus on various interests, from book clubs to hiking groups. Engaging in shared activities can lead to deeper connections and friendships.

- **Meetup Groups:** Utilize platforms like Meetup to find groups focused on women's health or social activities. This can be a great way to meet new people in your area.

How to Talk About Menopause with Family, Friends, and Co-Workers

Open communication is vital when discussing menopause, whether with family, friends, or colleagues. Here are some tips for effective communication:

1. Be Open and Honest

- **Share Your Experience:** Be honest about what you're experiencing. Sharing your symptoms and feelings can help others understand your situation better and provide the support you need.

- **Educate Others:** Many people may not be familiar with menopause or its effects. Use this opportunity to educate those around you about what you're going through.

2. Choose the Right Time and Place

- **Private Conversations:** Choose a private and comfortable setting to discuss menopause with close family and friends. This allows for a more open dialogue without distractions.

- **Professional Context:** When talking to co-workers or supervisors, consider discussing menopause during a one-on-one meeting or a suitable time when you can address concerns without interruptions.

3. Set Boundaries

- **Discuss Comfort Levels:** Make it clear what you're comfortable discussing and what you prefer to keep private. Setting boundaries helps manage expectations and fosters a respectful dialogue.

- **Encourage Questions:** Let your loved ones know that it's okay to ask questions if they want to understand your experiences better. This can foster a more supportive environment.

Menopause in the Workplace: Navigating Career and Health Challenges

Menopause can impact your professional life, and navigating this phase at work can be challenging. Here are strategies to help you address these issues:

1. Know Your Rights

- **Understand Workplace Policies:** Familiarize yourself with your employer's policies regarding health issues, workplace accommodations, and anti-discrimination laws. Knowing your rights can empower you to advocate for yourself.

- **Seek Accommodations:** If symptoms significantly affect your work performance, consider requesting accommodations such as flexible working hours, a comfortable workspace, or options to manage hot flashes.

2. Communicate with HR

- **Engage Human Resources:** If you feel comfortable, discuss your needs with your HR department. They can provide guidance on available resources and support options within the company.

- **Workplace Wellness Programs:** Inquire about workplace wellness initiatives that may offer resources, workshops, or support for women experiencing menopause.

3. Build a Support Network at Work

- **Connect with Colleagues:** Find co-workers who may be going through similar experiences. Building a network of support within your workplace can help normalize discussions about menopause and create a more understanding environment.

- **Share Resources:** If you come across helpful articles or resources about menopause, consider sharing them with colleagues. This can spark conversations and promote a culture of understanding.

Creating a Menopause-Friendly Community

Creating a supportive community for women experiencing menopause can significantly enhance the experience for everyone involved. Here are steps to foster such a community:

1. Start the Conversation

- **Initiate Discussions:** Organize informal gatherings, book clubs, or discussion groups focusing on menopause and women's health. Encourage open dialogue to create a comfortable space for sharing experiences.

- **Host Events:** Plan community events, such as workshops, health fairs, or seminars, to raise awareness about menopause and provide valuable information to women.

2. Collaborate with Local Organizations

- **Partner with Health Professionals:** Work with local healthcare providers, wellness centers, or community organizations to host educational events on menopause.

- **Engage with Nonprofits:** Collaborate with nonprofits focused on women's health to raise awareness, share resources, and create impactful programming.

3. Use Social Media

- **Online Communities:** Create or join online support groups or forums dedicated to menopause. These platforms allow for shared experiences and resources in a supportive environment.

- **Awareness Campaigns:** Use social media to share information, personal stories, and resources about menopause, helping to break the stigma and increase awareness within your community.

Building a strong support system during menopause is essential for navigating this transitional phase with confidence and grace. By connecting with other women, communicating openly with family and friends, addressing challenges in the workplace, and creating a menopause-friendly community, you can foster a supportive environment that enhances your experience. Remember, you are not alone in this journey—by reaching out and sharing your experiences, you empower yourself and others to thrive during this transformative time of life. Embrace the connections you make, and let them enrich your life as you move forward through menopause and beyond.

Chapter 15

Thriving in Midlife: Embracing the Wisdom Years

As you navigate the changes that come with menopause and move into the postmenopausal phase, it's essential to embrace this new chapter of life with confidence and purpose. Midlife is not a time to retreat or feel diminished; rather, it is an opportunity to celebrate your strength, wisdom, and accomplishments. In this chapter, we will explore the power of aging gracefully, the importance of celebrating your journey, inspiring stories from women who have thrived post-menopause, and how to find purpose in this life stage.

The Power of Aging Gracefully: Shifting Perspectives on Beauty and Worth

Aging is often viewed through a negative lens in our society, but it's time to shift that perspective and recognize the beauty and worth that come with age.

1. Redefining Beauty

- **Inner vs. Outer Beauty:** Acknowledge that true beauty comes from within. Emphasize qualities such as kindness, empathy, resilience, and confidence, which only deepen with life experience.

- **Media Representation:** Advocate for more diverse and realistic representations of aging in media and marketing. Support brands that celebrate women of all ages, recognizing that beauty is not confined to youth.

2. Embracing Your Unique Journey

- **Celebrate Individuality:** Embrace the unique experiences that shape you, including the challenges and triumphs of midlife. These experiences contribute to your identity and self-worth.

- **Shift in Perspective:** Practice gratitude for the wisdom and insights you have gained over the years. Focus on how far you've come rather than what you may have lost.

3. Cultivating a Positive Mindset

- **Affirmations and Positivity:** Use positive affirmations to cultivate a mindset that embraces aging. Remind yourself daily of your strengths and the value you bring to the world.

- **Mindfulness Practices:** Incorporate mindfulness and self-compassion practices into your daily routine. This can help you cultivate a more loving relationship with yourself as you age.

Celebrating Your Strength, Wisdom, and Accomplishments

Midlife is a time to celebrate your journey and recognize the strengths and wisdom you have gained.

1. Acknowledging Your Accomplishments

- **Reflect on Achievements:** Take time to reflect on your personal and professional achievements. Create a list of milestones you've reached, whether big or small, and celebrate each one.

- **Share Your Story:** Consider sharing your experiences with others. This can inspire and empower women who are navigating similar challenges.

2. Building Resilience

- **Resilience Through Challenges:** Recognize how past challenges have shaped your strength and resilience. Reflect on how you've overcome obstacles and how they have contributed to your character.

- **Lessons Learned:** Write about the lessons you've learned throughout your life. This practice can help you gain clarity on your journey and highlight the wisdom you possess.

3. Creating a Legacy

- **Document Your Journey:** Consider creating a journal, scrapbook, or blog to document your journey through midlife. This can serve as a reflection of your experiences and a legacy for future generations.

- **Mentorship and Guidance:** Offer your wisdom to younger women in your life. Consider mentoring or volunteering in programs that support young women, providing guidance based on your experiences.

Inspiring Stories from Women Who Have Thrived Post-Menopause

Hearing stories from other women who have thrived after menopause can be incredibly inspiring. Here are some examples:

1. The Artist

- **Rediscovering Passion:** A woman in her 60s who spent most of her life caring for others decided to pursue her lifelong passion for painting after her children left home. Through her art, she found a voice and community, leading to a successful exhibition showcasing her work.

2. The Entrepreneur

- **Starting a New Venture:** After retiring from a long career in corporate finance, a woman in her 50s started a business that aligned with her passion for health and wellness. Her venture has not only brought her joy but also allowed her to help others on their wellness journeys.

3. The Activist

- **Advocating for Change:** A woman who experienced health challenges during menopause became an advocate for women's health issues. Through her activism, she raised awareness about menopause, pushing for better resources and support for women in her community.

4. The Traveler

- **Exploring the World:** After menopause, a woman decided to fulfill her dream of traveling the world. She visited different countries, embraced new cultures, and documented her adventures, inspiring others to step outside their comfort zones.

Finding Purpose: How to Make the Most of This Life Stage

Midlife is an excellent time to reassess your goals and find purpose in your life.

1. Pursuing Passions

- **Identify What Excites You:** Take time to explore what truly excites you. Whether it's a hobby, a cause, or a career change, pursuing your passions can bring renewed energy and joy to your life.

- **Try New Things:** Don't hesitate to step outside your comfort zone and try new activities. Joining classes, workshops, or clubs can open doors to new interests and friendships.

2. Setting Meaningful Goals

- **Short-Term vs. Long-Term Goals:** Reflect on both short-term and long-term goals. Consider what you want to achieve in the next few months, as well as the dreams you want to pursue in the coming years.

- **SMART Goals:** Use the SMART criteria (Specific, Measurable, Achievable, Relevant, Time-bound) to create clear goals that are actionable and meaningful to you.

3. Giving Back

- **Volunteer Work:** Find ways to give back to your community through volunteer work. Whether it's mentoring, tutoring, or supporting local organizations, helping others can provide a deep sense of fulfillment.

- **Involvement in Causes:** Get involved in causes you are passionate about. Whether it's environmental issues, women's rights, or health advocacy, contributing to a cause can reignite your sense of purpose.

Midlife is a powerful and transformative time filled with opportunities to embrace your wisdom and experience. By shifting your perspective on aging, celebrating your strengths and accomplishments, learning from the inspiring stories of others, and actively seeking purpose, you can thrive in this new chapter of life. Embrace the wisdom years as a time of growth, renewal, and empowerment, and remember that your journey is unique and

valuable. As you move forward, let your experiences shape the next chapter, enriching your

life and the lives of those around you.

Chapter 15

Thriving in Midlife: Embracing the Wisdom Years

As you navigate the changes that come with menopause and move into the postmenopausal phase, it's essential to embrace this new chapter of life with confidence and purpose. Midlife is not a time to retreat or feel diminished; rather, it is an opportunity to celebrate your strength, wisdom, and accomplishments. In this chapter, we will explore the power of aging gracefully, the importance of celebrating your journey, inspiring stories from women who have thrived post-menopause, and how to find purpose in this life stage.

The Power of Aging Gracefully: Shifting Perspectives on Beauty and Worth

Aging is often viewed through a negative lens in our society, but it's time to shift that perspective and recognize the beauty and worth that come with age.

1. Redefining Beauty

- **Inner vs. Outer Beauty:** Acknowledge that true beauty comes from within. Emphasize qualities such as kindness, empathy, resilience, and confidence, which only deepen with life experience.

- **Media Representation:** Advocate for more diverse and realistic representations of aging in media and marketing. Support brands that celebrate women of all ages, recognizing that beauty is not confined to youth.

2. Embracing Your Unique Journey

- **Celebrate Individuality:** Embrace the unique experiences that shape you, including the challenges and triumphs of midlife. These experiences contribute to your identity and self-worth.

- **Shift in Perspective:** Practice gratitude for the wisdom and insights you have gained over the years. Focus on how far you've come rather than what you may have lost.

3. Cultivating a Positive Mindset

- **Affirmations and Positivity:** Use positive affirmations to cultivate a mindset that embraces aging. Remind yourself daily of your strengths and the value you bring to the world.

- **Mindfulness Practices:** Incorporate mindfulness and self-compassion practices into your daily routine. This can help you cultivate a more loving relationship with yourself as you age.

Celebrating Your Strength, Wisdom, and Accomplishments

Midlife is a time to celebrate your journey and recognize the strengths and wisdom you have gained.

1. Acknowledging Your Accomplishments

- **Reflect on Achievements:** Take time to reflect on your personal and professional achievements. Create a list of milestones you've reached, whether big or small, and celebrate each one.

- **Share Your Story:** Consider sharing your experiences with others. This can inspire and empower women who are navigating similar challenges.

2. Building Resilience

- **Resilience Through Challenges:** Recognize how past challenges have shaped your strength and resilience. Reflect on how you've overcome obstacles and how they have contributed to your character.

- **Lessons Learned:** Write about the lessons you've learned throughout your life. This practice can help you gain clarity on your journey and highlight the wisdom you possess.

3. Creating a Legacy

- **Document Your Journey:** Consider creating a journal, scrapbook, or blog to document your journey through midlife. This can serve as a reflection of your experiences and a legacy for future generations.

- **Mentorship and Guidance:** Offer your wisdom to younger women in your life. Consider mentoring or volunteering in programs that support young women, providing guidance based on your experiences.

Inspiring Stories from Women Who Have Thrived Post-Menopause

Hearing stories from other women who have thrived after menopause can be incredibly inspiring. Here are some examples:

1. The Artist

- **Rediscovering Passion:** A woman in her 60s who spent most of her life caring for others decided to pursue her lifelong passion for painting after her children left home. Through her art, she found a voice and community, leading to a successful exhibition showcasing her work.

2. The Entrepreneur

- **Starting a New Venture:** After retiring from a long career in corporate finance, a woman in her 50s started a business that aligned with her passion for health and wellness. Her venture has not only brought her joy but also allowed her to help others on their wellness journeys.

3. The Activist

- **Advocating for Change:** A woman who experienced health challenges during menopause became an advocate for women's health issues. Through her activism, she raised awareness about menopause, pushing for better resources and support for women in her community.

4. The Traveler

- **Exploring the World:** After menopause, a woman decided to fulfill her dream of traveling the world. She visited different countries, embraced new cultures, and documented her adventures, inspiring others to step outside their comfort zones.

Finding Purpose: How to Make the Most of This Life Stage

Midlife is an excellent time to reassess your goals and find purpose in your life.

1. Pursuing Passions

- **Identify What Excites You:** Take time to explore what truly excites you. Whether it's a hobby, a cause, or a career change, pursuing your passions can bring renewed energy and joy to your life.

- **Try New Things:** Don't hesitate to step outside your comfort zone and try new activities. Joining classes, workshops, or clubs can open doors to new interests and friendships.

2. Setting Meaningful Goals

- **Short-Term vs. Long-Term Goals:** Reflect on both short-term and long-term goals. Consider what you want to achieve in the next few months, as well as the dreams you want to pursue in the coming years.

- **SMART Goals:** Use the SMART criteria (Specific, Measurable, Achievable, Relevant, Time-bound) to create clear goals that are actionable and meaningful to you.

3. Giving Back

- **Volunteer Work:** Find ways to give back to your community through volunteer work. Whether it's mentoring, tutoring, or supporting local organizations, helping others can provide a deep sense of fulfillment.

- **Involvement in Causes:** Get involved in causes you are passionate about. Whether it's environmental issues, women's rights, or health advocacy, contributing to a cause can reignite your sense of purpose.

Midlife is a powerful and transformative time filled with opportunities to embrace your wisdom and experience. By shifting your perspective on aging, celebrating your strengths and accomplishments, learning from the inspiring stories of others, and actively seeking purpose, you can thrive in this new chapter of life. Embrace the wisdom years as a time of growth, renewal, and empowerment, and remember that your journey is unique and valuable. As you move forward, let your experiences shape the next chapter, enriching your life and the lives of those around you.

Lifestyle Modifications

In navigating the challenges of menopause, lifestyle modifications play a crucial role in managing symptoms and improving overall health. This chapter focuses on dietary choices and exercise strategies that can empower women during this transition, helping them maintain their well-being and quality of life.

Diet and Nutrition

1. Importance of a Balanced Diet

A balanced diet is essential for maintaining optimal health during menopause. Proper nutrition can help alleviate some menopause symptoms, support hormone balance, and reduce the risk of chronic diseases.

- **Key Components of a Balanced Diet:**
  - **Fruits and Vegetables:** Aim for at least five servings per day. These foods are rich in vitamins, minerals, antioxidants, and fiber, which are vital for overall health.
    - *Examples:* Berries (antioxidants), leafy greens (calcium), and citrus fruits (vitamin C).
  - **Whole Grains:** Incorporate whole grains for sustained energy and to aid digestion.
    - *Examples:* Brown rice, quinoa, oatmeal, and whole wheat bread.

- Lean Proteins: Essential for muscle maintenance, especially during a time when metabolism may slow down.

    - *Examples:* Skinless poultry, fish, beans, legumes, and tofu.

- **Healthy Fats:** Support heart health and hormone production.

    - *Examples:* Avocado, nuts, seeds, olive oil, and fatty fish like salmon (rich in omega-3 fatty acids).

2. Foods That Help Balance Hormones

Certain foods contain compounds that can mimic estrogen in the body, known as phytoestrogens, which may help alleviate some menopause symptoms.

- **Phytoestrogen-Rich Foods:**

    - **Soy Products:** Tofu, tempeh, edamame, and soy milk are excellent sources of isoflavones, a type of phytoestrogen.

    - **Flaxseeds:** High in lignans, flaxseeds can help balance hormones. Ground flaxseeds can be added to smoothies, oatmeal, or yogurt.

    - **Legumes:** Beans, lentils, and chickpeas are not only sources of protein but also contain phytoestrogens that can aid in hormone balance.

    - **Whole Grains:** Barley, oats, and whole grain bread provide fiber and phytoestrogens, contributing to hormone regulation.

    - **Fruits and Vegetables:** Certain varieties, such as carrots, apples, and pomegranates, contain phytoestrogens that support hormonal health.

3. Additional Nutritional Considerations

- **Calcium and Vitamin D:**

    - As women approach menopause, the risk of osteoporosis increases. Calcium and vitamin D are vital for bone health.

    - *Sources of Calcium:* Dairy products, leafy greens, and fortified plant-based milk.

- *Sources of Vitamin D:* Fatty fish, egg yolks, and fortified foods, along with sunlight exposure.

- **Hydration:**

    - Staying well-hydrated helps with overall health and can alleviate symptoms like dryness and fatigue. Aim for at least 8-10 glasses of water a day, adjusting for activity level and climate.

Exercise

1. Importance of Regular Physical Activity

Regular exercise is crucial during menopause for various reasons:

- **Weight Management:** Helps counteract weight gain that often accompanies hormonal changes.

- **Mood Enhancement:** Physical activity stimulates the production of endorphins, improving mood and reducing anxiety and depression.

- **Bone Health:** Weight-bearing exercises can strengthen bones, reducing the risk of osteoporosis.

- **Cardiovascular Health:** Regular exercise supports heart health, which is especially important post-menopause due to increased heart disease risk.

2. Recommended Types of Exercise

Incorporating a variety of exercise types can help address different health concerns associated with menopause.

Aerobic Exercise

- **Benefits:** Improves cardiovascular fitness, helps maintain a healthy weight, and boosts mood.

- **Recommendations:** Aim for at least 150 minutes of moderate-intensity aerobic exercise per week.

    - *Examples:* Walking, cycling, swimming, and dancing.

Strength Training

- **Benefits:** Builds muscle mass, enhances metabolism, and strengthens bones.

- **Recommendations:** Include strength training exercises at least two days a week.

    o *Examples:* Weight lifting, resistance band exercises, or body-weight exercises (like push-ups and squats).

Flexibility and Balance Exercises

- **Benefits:** Improves range of motion, reduces the risk of falls, and enhances overall mobility.

- **Recommendations:** Incorporate stretching and balance exercises at least two to three times a week.

    o *Examples:* Yoga, Pilates, tai chi, and simple stretching routines.

3. Creating an Exercise Routine

To maximize the benefits of exercise during menopause, consider the following tips:

- **Set Realistic Goals:** Start with achievable goals and gradually increase intensity and duration.

- **Find Activities You Enjoy:** Engaging in activities you enjoy will make it easier to stay motivated and consistent.

- **Mix It Up:** Variety in workouts can prevent boredom and provide a well-rounded fitness regimen.

- **Listen to Your Body:** Pay attention to how your body feels during and after exercise, adjusting intensity as needed, especially if experiencing symptoms like fatigue or joint pain.

Lifestyle modifications involving diet and exercise are powerful tools for managing menopause symptoms and enhancing overall health. By focusing on a balanced diet rich in hormone-supporting foods and incorporating regular physical activity, women can navigate this transition with resilience and vitality. Taking proactive steps towards wellness not only alleviates symptoms but also contributes to long-term health benefits, empowering women to thrive during and beyond menopause.

Conclusion

Cool, Calm, and Empowered

As we reach the end of our journey through the complexities of menopause, it's essential to reflect on the empowering insights and tools that have been shared throughout this guide. Menopause can be a time of significant change, but it can also be an opportunity for personal growth, self-discovery, and renewed strength. Here, we summarize key takeaways and encourage you to embrace this new chapter of your life with confidence and grace.

A Final Word on Thriving Through Menopause

Menopause is not merely a medical transition; it is a transformative phase that offers women a chance to redefine themselves and their lives. By understanding the symptoms, embracing lifestyle modifications, and cultivating a strong support system, you can navigate this period with resilience. Remember, it's perfectly normal to experience a range of emotions and physical changes; what matters most is how you respond to these changes.

- **Empowerment Through Knowledge:** Knowledge is your ally. By learning about menopause, you can debunk myths and reduce anxiety about the unknown.

- **Self-Care is Essential:** Prioritize self-care, including physical, emotional, and mental well-being. The strategies outlined in this guide are designed to help you thrive, not just survive.

- **Embrace Humor and Positivity:** Maintaining a sense of humor can lighten the experience of menopause. Laughing at the absurdities of life can foster resilience and make challenges feel more manageable.

Looking Forward: The Next Chapter of Your Life

As you move forward, consider this time as the beginning of a new adventure. With the challenges of menopause behind you, you have the opportunity to embrace newfound freedom and pursue your passions.

- **Personal Growth:** Use this time to explore interests you may have set aside or discover new hobbies that ignite your enthusiasm. Whether it's traveling, learning a new skill, or volunteering, now is the time to invest in yourself.

- **Reinvention:** Many women find that menopause sparks a desire to reinvent themselves. Whether it's changing careers, starting a business, or focusing on personal development, view this period as a chance to align your life with your evolving values and goals.

Resources for Further Reading and Support

As you continue your journey through menopause and beyond, consider seeking out additional resources for support and information. Here are some recommendations:

- **Books:**

    o *The Wisdom of Menopause* by Christiane Northrup

    o *Menopause Confidential* by Tara Allmen

    o *The Menopause Manifesto* by Dr. Jen Gunter

- **Websites and Online Communities:**

    o **North American Menopause Society (NAMS):** www.menopause.org

    o **Menopause Matters:** www.menopausematters.co.uk

    o **Reddit's r/Menopause Community:** A supportive forum for sharing experiences and advice.

- **Support Groups:**

    o Consider joining local or online support groups for women experiencing menopause. Connecting with others can provide comfort and solidarity during this transition.

Acknowledgements and Thanks

This guide would not have been possible without the contributions of countless women who have bravely shared their experiences, insights, and wisdom. Your voices matter, and your strength inspires others.

Thank you to healthcare professionals dedicated to supporting women's health, who provide invaluable information and resources for managing menopause. Your commitment to women's well-being is deeply appreciated.

To all the readers: your willingness to engage with this journey is commendable. Remember, menopause is just one chapter in a rich tapestry of life. Embrace the changes, celebrate your strengths, and move forward with confidence, knowing that you are cool, calm, and empowered to thrive. Here's to the next exciting chapter of your life!

References

1. Allmen, T. (2017). *Menopause confidential: A doctor reveals the 411 on popular therapies and treatments*. Da Capo Lifelong Books.

2. American College of Obstetricians and Gynecologists. (2020). *Menopause*. Retrieved from https://www.acog.org/clinical/clinical-guidance/committee-opinion/articles/2020/09/menopause

3. American Menopause Society. (n.d.). *Menopause*. Retrieved from https://www.menopause.org

4. Bradshaw, M. (2019). *The menopause handbook: A guide for women*. Hachette UK.

5. Brody, J. E. (2019). Hot flashes? Here's what you need to know. *The New York Times*. Retrieved from https://www.nytimes.com

6. Christiane Northrup, M. D. (2010). *The wisdom of menopause: Creating physical and emotional health during the change*. Hay House.

7. Gunter, J. (2021). *The menopause manifesto: Own your health with facts and feminism*. HarperCollins.

8. Harlow, S. D., & Gass, M. (2020). Executive summary of the Stages of Reproductive Aging Workshop + 10: Addressing the unfinished agenda of women's health during the menopause transition. *Menopause*, 27(8), 847-856. https://doi.org/10.1097/GME.0000000000001607

9. Kahn, J. R. (2017). *Menopause: The one-stop guide*. Hachette UK.

10. Kuehner, C. (2017). Why do women suffer from depression more than men? *The Lancet Psychiatry*, 4(2), 146-158. https://doi.org/10.1016/S2215-0366(16)30399-4

11. Lee, J. C. (2018). Nutritional management of menopause. *Nutritional Reviews*, 76(9), 644-659. https://doi.org/10.1093/nutrit/nuy037

12. Levey, J. A., & Ross, J. S. (2018). Menopause management: An evidence-based approach. *American Family Physician*, 98(3), 162-169.

13. Lichtenstein, A. H., & Appel, L. J. (2021). AHA/ACC/WHO scientific statement: Healthy dietary patterns. *Circulation*, 143(1), e69-e86. https://doi.org/10.1161/CIR.0000000000000832

14. McKinlay, S. M., & Brambilla, D. J. (2019). The role of hormonal changes in the onset of menopause symptoms. *Journal of Women's Health*, 28(7), 951-958. https://doi.org/10.1089/jwh.2018.7004

15. Miller, J. A. (2018). *Menopause: A comprehensive guide to health and well-being*. WestBow Press.

16. North American Menopause Society. (2021). *The menopause transition*. Retrieved from https://www.menopause.org/for-women/menopause

17. Reddy, S., & Brinton, R. D. (2019). Hormone therapy: A new perspective on estrogen and the brain. *Endocrinology*, 160(4), 1039-1048. https://doi.org/10.1210/en.2018-01306

18. Ross, A. M., & Yandle, M. (2020). Managing menopausal symptoms in women with a history of breast cancer: A review. *Current Oncology Reports*, 22(12), 104. https://doi.org/10.1007/s11912-020-00988-0

19. Stuenkel, C. A., et al. (2015). *Treatment of menopause-associated vasomotor symptoms: An endocrine society clinical practice guideline. The Journal of Clinical Endocrinology & Metabolism*, 100(6), 3968-3992. https://doi.org/10.1210/jc.2015-2236

20. Sweeney, E. E. (2021). *The menopause diet: A practical guide to changing your diet for health and vitality*. Clearview Publishing.

21. Terauchi, M., & Nakano, Y. (2018). The relationship between menopause and cognitive function: A systematic review. *Neuropsychology Review*, 28(4), 335-353. https://doi.org/10.1007/s11065-018-9404-7

22. United States Department of Health & Human Services. (2019). *Menopause: A health guide for women*. Retrieved from https://www.womenshealth.gov

23. Utian, W. H. (2005). The Menopause: A Comprehensive Approach. *Menopause*, 12(3), 400-412. https://doi.org/10.1097/01.gme.0000170953.09943.66

24. van der Molen, H. J., et al. (2019). The relationship between menopause and depression: A systematic review. *Psychoneuroendocrinology*, 101, 159-167. https://doi.org/10.1016/j.psyneuen.2018.10.019

25. Vitzthum, V. J. (2019). Hormonal changes in menopause: Implications for health. *Annual Review of Anthropology*, 48, 151-167. https://doi.org/10.1146/annurev-anthro-102018-023210

26. Wysowski, D. K., & Swartz, L. (2017). Hormone therapy for menopause symptoms: A review of the evidence. *American Family Physician*, 96(8), 543-549.

27. Yamaguchi, T., & Ryu, S. (2020). Effects of exercise on menopause-related symptoms: A systematic review. *Menopause*, 27(6), 666-674. https://doi.org/10.1097/GME.0000000000001441

28. Zhuang, C., & Wang, Y. (2018). A review of complementary and alternative medicine for menopause symptoms: Safety and effectiveness. *Journal of Clinical Endocrinology & Metabolism*, 103(10), 3718-3727. https://doi.org/10.1210/jc.2018-01023

29. Howard, L. J., & Martin, J. M. (2020). *Menopause: An issue of clinical relevance in women's health*. Journal of Women's Health, 29(1), 1-5. https://doi.org/10.1089/jwh.2020.2834

30. Speroff, L., & Fritz, M. A. (2011). *Clinical gynecologic endocrinology and infertility* (8th ed.). Lippincott Williams & Wilkins.

31. Maclennan, A. H., et al. (2004). A systematic review of the effectiveness of hormone replacement therapy in menopause. *British Journal of Obstetrics and Gynaecology*, 111(8), 694-702. https://doi.org/10.1111/j.1471-0528.2004.00133.x

32. The North American Menopause Society. (2020). *Menopause practice: A clinician's guide* (5th ed.). The North American Menopause Society.

33. Kagan, R. (2021). *Menopause and your mental health: How to cope with changes during the transition*. New Harbinger Publications.

34. Beck, A. T., & Hauser, K. (2019). *Cognitive therapy of depression*. Guilford Press.

35. Minkin, M. J. (2019). *Menopause 101: A simple guide to the facts and treatments*. Health Communications.

36. Davis, S. R., et al. (2019). The menopause: A time of change. *The Lancet*, 394(10205), 303-316. https://doi.org/10.1016/S0140-6736(19)31811-5

37. Melby, M. K. (2020). *Menopause: A woman's transition through midlife*. University of Minnesota Press.

38. Nelson, H. D., et al. (2012). Hormone therapy for the management of menopause-related symptoms: A systematic review. *Annals of Internal Medicine*, 157(2), 104-113. https://doi.org/10.7326/0003-4819-157-2-201207170-00008

39. Shapiro, G. K., et al. (2018). What do women want in menopause care? *BMC Women's Health*, 18(1), 48. https://doi.org/10.1186/s12905-018-0543-4

40. Sowers, M. F., & Crandall, C. J. (2019). Menopause and aging. *The Journal of Clinical Endocrinology & Metabolism*, 104(12), 5767-5777. https://doi.org/10.1210/jc.2019-00409